Pharmaceutical
Project Management

Pharmaceutical Project Management
Second Edition

edited by
Tony Kennedy
Trigen Ltd
London, UK

informa
healthcare

New York   London

Informa Healthcare USA, Inc.
52 Vanderbilt Avenue
New York, NY 10017

© 2008 by Informa Healthcare USA, Inc.
Informa Healthcare is an Informa business

No claim to original U.S. Government works
Printed in the United States of America on acid-free paper
10 9 8 7 6 5 4 3 2 1

International Standard Book Number-10: 0-8493-4024-1 (Hardcover)
International Standard Book Number-13: 978-0-8493-4024-6 (Hardcover)

Library of Congress Cataloging-in-Publication Data

Pharmaceutical project management / edited by Tony Kennedy. – 2nd ed.
   p. ; cm. – (Drugs and the pharmaceutical sciences; 182)
   Includes bibliographical references and index.
   ISBN-13: 978-0-8493-4024-6 (hb : alk. paper)
   ISBN-10: 0-8493-4024-1 (hb : alk. paper)
   1. Pharmaceutical industry.   2. Project management.   I. Kennedy, Tony, 1948–.
   [DNLM: 1. Drug Industry – organization & administration.   2. Drug Evaluation.   3. Research – organization & administration.   QV 736 P53617 2008]

   RS192.P465 2008
   338.4′76151 – dc22   2007044284

For Corporate Sales and Reprint Permissions call 212-520-2700 or write to: Sales Department, 52 Vanderbilt, 16th floor, New York, NY 10017

Visit the Informa Web site at
www.informa.com

and the Informa Healthcare Web site at
www.informahealthcare.com

Preface

This second edition of *Pharmaceutical Project Management* is published one decade after the first edition. What has changed over the past decade in drug development? Actually, a lot. The move to outsourcing has intensified and the successful management of relationships between sponsor and contractor is recognized to be a critical competence. Productivity as measured by the number of new medicines marketed each year declined dramatically in spite of the optimism about new science and technology. Despite spending more on research and development we are not getting any smarter in picking out the medicines from the molecules. Drug development times for the fewer drugs taken to market were faster and regulatory authorities reduced approval times. We also witnessed a change in the landscape as faltering pharmaceutical giants broke up the colossus into potentially nimbler, smaller therapeutic units in discovery and development.

What does it mean for pharma project management today? It means that companies cannot rest on their laurels, but have to continuously find better ways to develop drugs. Decision making clearly needs to be better. Novel drug development "projects" actually are a series of projects subsumed under a strategic intent. Sequential investments are made. The quality of the planning, execution, review, and decision making for each investment cycle will set apart future winners from "also rans." Speed to market will always be important. As development times have been reduced, the chemistry, manufacturing, and controls team increasingly is under pressure to deliver to demanding schedules. Most companies now have a mixed model in which a significant proportion of "development parts" are outsourced. The effective management of contracted development is a central theme in future drug development project management. The second edition has been designed to focus on the strategic and operational strategies that will enable companies to compete effectively in this new landscape of drug development.

Chapter 1 reviews strategy at the project level. It discusses the objectives of each development phase and why projects fail. The strategic tools and their uses are described. The decision-making process for project progression or termination is critically examined. Project development strategies are cited.

Chapter 2 describes the aims of portfolio management and the tools and the processes that can be used. These include tools to optimize the portfolio with respect to time, to risk, or to resource and return. Financial modeling including modeling uncertainty is explored. The different perspectives of customers and practitioners are considered. Finally the authors provide a pragmatic and realistic account of how portfolios can be managed, recognizing the diversity of the company needs.

Chapter 3 systemically describes how project plans are created. The steps in the planning process, the nature of the activities, establishing the Gantt, optimizing the plan, and managing the planning process are described. Planning systems are described.

Chapters 4 and 5 focus on chemistry, manufacturing, and controls. Chapter 4 describes the nature of the chemistry, manufacturing, and controls development work and the challenges and strategic options to achieve success and is written by the leader of the chemistry, manufacturing, and controls teams that brought Sequinavir and Tamiflu rapidly to market. The perspective of a contract company working with pharma is described in Chapter 5 which emphasizes the importance of establishing a mature relationship if project success is to be achieved. Differences between custom, contract, and toll manufacturing are explained. Information flow, risk management, and quality are the key challenges that contract manufacturers have to successfully address.

Chapter 6 makes a robust assessment of the state of clinical trial project management in a broad ranging text. Chapter 7 reviews the roles and responsibilities of regulatory sub-teams and how they work with the central project team. Regulatory project management practice is discussed.

Chapter 8 offers a provocative review about teams in describing how they operate in the real world, with ideas as to how they can improve their effectiveness.

In Chapter 9, the variety of outsourcing models that can be used are explained with expert evaluation of the challenges of each and the management strategies best employed. Specific examples are cited that give real world insight.

The concluding Chapter 10 describes the scope of the responsibilities of a project management function at project, portfolio, and pharma support levels. The skills and competencies that are required are considered and suggestions made on how these may be acquired.

Tony Kennedy

Contents

Contributors

Kevin Bilyard   Nine-TZ Healthcare Ventures, Wilmslow, Cheshire, U.K.

Jon Court   Fulcrum Pharma Developments Ltd., Hemel Hempstead, U.K.

Mark Fowler   Strategic Sourcing & Procurement, Amgen Inc, Thousand Oaks, California, U.S.A.

Tony Kennedy   Trigen Ltd., London, U.K.

Dieter Krimmer   Rapid Pharma Development GmbH, Unteraegeri, Switzerland

Carl A. Kutzbach   Previously Bayer AG, Wuppertal, Germany

Des Markland   Decanalysis Ltd., Congleton, Cheshire, U.K.

Les Rose   Pharmavision Consulting Ltd., West Harnham, Salisbury, U.K.

Carole Strong   EXRO Pharma Solutions Ltd., Hertfordshire, U.K.

Lukas M. J. von Hippel   AllessaChemie GmbH, Frankfurt am Main, Germany

Sylvia Walker   EXRO Pharma Solutions Ltd., Hertfordshire, U.K.

Nicholas Wells   Independent Pharma Consultants, Kent, U.K.

Ralph White   PPMLD Ltd., London, U.K.

1

Strategic Project Management at the Project Level

Tony Kennedy
Trigen Ltd., London, U.K.

INTRODUCTION

This chapter is about the drug development strategy considered at the level of individual projects. There are a range of questions to be considered for drug development projects. How are projects brought to market quickly? How do we decide which projects are likely winners and losers? How can we avoid wasted expenditure on projects? What can be done to get the best return on the projects that make it to the market? How do we organize ourselves to develop drugs effectively? These questions are addressed in the context of the broad strategic challenges we face in developing new drugs. Good strategies can be found by understanding the inherent risks in developing drugs, when these risks are encountered, and how sensible risk-management strategies can be implemented. Drug development is a business and, as with all businesses, must be profitable for it to flourish in the future. The fundamentals of any business depend upon getting a worthwhile return on investment. For the innovator pharmaceutical industry, a critical determinant of profitability lies in the limited time exclusivity granted by governments to companies through the patent system. While much criticized, the patent system powers investments in new sciences and new medicines. Without it, innovation would wither on the vine because innovator companies would have no chance to recoup investments in a world where commodity substitution has never been faster. This chapter attempts to characterize the drug development process, and in doing so identify strategies that can be used to conduct drug development in a business-like manner. The drug development process is not just about gaining

1

marketing authorization—though that is a major achievement. It is also about providing the best evidence at the right time to support the product-labeling that the product deserves and the evidence and information that enables a company to reach and persuade the various "customers" for the drug—those who write the clinical practice guidelines, those who decide reimbursement, and those who decide regional and local drug-prescribing practice. If all the deciders in the drug prescription decision chain are not convinced, then the drug will not be fully adopted and the commercial potential will not be realized.

The first section describes the "terrain" of drug development, the phases of drug development, and the key objectives of these phases. The high rate of failure of development projects is highlighted and the reasons for the failures are discussed. Since most projects fail, it is obvious that recognizing nonviable projects early is important so that money and resources can be diverted to projects offering more promise. The quality of decision making is clearly critically important.

The second section discusses how project teams select a development strategy for their project and how they capture it and communicate it within the company. It explores the decision-making process for assessing project viability from acceptance of projects into the development pipeline through the phases of development to registration, launch, postlaunch lifecycle management (LCM), and an ultimate disinvestment decision. This is reviewed from the perspectives of the project team, functional departments, and senior management.

The third section considers what can be done to maximize the commercial return for those rare "gold nuggets," projects that are both technically and commercially viable. Good strategies are needed to ensure that the full value of the project is realized and in this section, strategies to optimize the proprietary position, clinical and regulatory strategy, commercial and pharmacoeconomic strategy, and speed-to-market strategy are considered.

THE TERRAIN OF DRUG DEVELOPMENT

Phases of Drug Development

Drugs are developed over many years. Drug development usually follows a well-defined sequence (refer, however, to the "Speed-to-Market Strategy" section below). Drug development is a highly regulated and controlled environment in which activities are invariably conducted to defined standards and data requirements are prescribed so that it is possible for regulatory agencies to challenge the adequacy of the data submitted by companies to gain marketing approval. All projects are unique and in the following description the author "generalizes" in describing some key activities conducted in each development phase. Table 1 summarizes the six major phases of drug development that follow on from a decision to progress a molecule from discovery into development. Chapter 3 describes the scheduling of the key development:

Table 1 Key Project Activities During the Major Drug Development Phases for a Chronic Oral Drug Therapy

Key activities in phases of drug development	Preclinical	Phase 1	Phase 2	Phase 3	Registration	Life cycle management
Primary objectives of phase	To establish that a drug merits progression into human clinical testing	To establish that a drug merits progression into patient trials	To characterize a dose-response relationship for efficacy and safety	To provide pivotal trial evidence for efficacy and safety in chronic dosing	To secure registration approval for the intended product label	To maximize the commercial return for the product
We own the product	New patent applications (new salt forms, API crystal forms) filed	Formulation patents filed	Process patents filed; Trademark applications submitted	Patents filed for new clinical uses of the drug	Application for regulatory exclusivity submitted	New manufacturing process patents filed; New formulation patents filed; New indication patents filed
The product forms are viable	API scaled up to 5–10 kg Phase 1 dose form(s) made and short-term stability analysis done	API scaled up to 25–50 kg Tablets/capsules made at doses for phase 2 trial; Stability trial to cover phase 2 trial performed	Synthesis optimized and route "frozen" to supply phase 3 clinical trials/carcinogenicity studies	Representative manufacturing batches of the Tablets/capsules made; Extended stability trials run	Compilation of CMC dossier done; Progression initiation of product line extensions performed; Manufacture of launch batches started	Investment in API cost reduction done; Development of new product forms to support new indications started; Consumer marketing-driven product innovations undertaken
The product is "fit for use" (benefit/risk)	Short-term (up to 28 days) animal studies to define safety at exposure levels and above expected clinical exposure performed	Single dose "first in man" study done; Multiple-dose study done; Effect of food on oral drug absorption assessed; Drug interaction studies performed	Dose-finding studies in patients performed; Long-term animal safety studies (6/9 mo in rat/dog) progressed	Pivotal efficacy studies cf comparators done; Safety in extended dosing (to patients 12 mo) determined; Carcinogenicity trials ongoing	Integrated summaries of efficacy and safety prepared; Label claims finalized; Phase 3b new indication trials initiated	Postmarketing regulatory commitment studies done; Phase 4 marketing clinical trials including global and regional trials performed; Phase 4 postmarketing surveillance conducted

Abbreviations: API, active pharmaceutical ingredient; CMC, chemistry, manufacturing and controls.

1. Preclinical development seeks to provide adequate information to justify the safe first administration of a new drug to humans. It typically includes manufacture of sufficient drug substance (the active pharmaceutical ingredient, API), development of analytical methods to enable assessment of the purity of the API, and its purity in the drug product in short-term storage conditions. A program of toxicology and pharmacology will be completed to allow assessment of doses of the drug that can reasonably be tested on human volunteers. The level of drug exposure achieved in the toxicology studies will be determined and related to planned clinical exposure levels. Any findings from the toxicology and pharmacology studies will be carefully assessed to decide if the drug can, with reasonable safety, be administered to volunteers and to ensure close monitoring of potential clinical symptoms related to preclinical findings. Typically, this phase of development takes 9 to 15 months and may cost £1.5 million to £3 million.

2. Phase 1 development is focused upon demonstrating the safety and tolerability of the drug in volunteers and characterizing the pharmacokinetics of the drug in humans. Phase 1 studies should provide sufficient information to support advancing the drug into patient trials. Phase 1 volunteer studies are conducted in dedicated units, which allow for very close safety monitoring of patients. The first-in-human study generally involves a dose escalation from small doses. Guidelines for Phase 1 Clinical Trials have been published in 2007 by the Association of the British Pharmaceutical Industry and provide an excellent summary including discussion of the selection of dose for first-in-human studies (1). Often phase 1 clinical studies will include a single-dose first-in-man study and then a multiple-does study (e.g., seven-day dosing), which enables a dose regimen to be defined which in turn provides an appropriate systemic drug concentration to support the efficacy of the drug. An effect of food study on pharmacokinetics is often carried out so that recommendations can be made about the timing of drug dosing in relation to meal times for the planned phase 2 trials. Drug interaction studies may also be conducted so that commonly used comedications in the planned patient group can be checked to see if their performance or the performance of the new drug is modified. In some therapeutic areas, it is possible to get valuable efficacy data in phase 1. For example, a flu challenge study can be conducted in volunteers. While the clinical studies are ongoing, a range of other activities in drug synthesis route optimization, analytical development, formulation studies, toxicology, and studies of the drug handling in animal species and in vitro with human tissues will be progressed. Phase 1 may take 10 to 15 months to complete depending on the needed studies and may cost £2 million to £4 million.

3. Phase 2 development focuses on gaining initial information on the safety of the drug in patients and evaluating the dose–response relationship in patients to justify the selection of appropriate dose(s) regimen that will later be tested in the phase 3 pivotal trials. The clinical protocol for the phase 2 study will define the patient type to be studied and the clinical end points that will be measured to define the efficacy of the drug. Often three or four dose regimens

will be tested based upon a review of phase 1 data and the preclinical in vitro and in vivo data. In some therapeutic areas, useful "markers of activity" may be measured in phase 1 or phase 2a trials, which would assist in the selection of doses. The size of the phase 2 dose-finding trial will be influenced by the nature of the clinical end point and the number of patients that will be required to be studied to provide a reliable estimate of efficacy and the potential to discriminate between the dose regimens of different drugs. The duration and cost of phase 2 trials may differ considerably between different clinical indications. For example, a phase 2 trial for a drug being studied against an end point for which a strong and consistent treatment effect is predicted may require only 25 patients per dose group and so a 100-patient study may be adequate to define a dose–response relationship. In contrast, a drug, which is added onto other baseline therapies and for which a small incremental treatment effect is predicted and where inherent variability in the end point is high, may require a 1500-patient phase 2 trial. Drug regulators will look for evidence that the dose regimen recommended for phase 3 can be justified from the phase 2 trial results. For example, the mid-dose of a phase 2 trial may be recommended because no significant improvement in efficacy was offered by the high dose studied. Alternatively, the mid-dose is recommended since the high dose provided marginal increase in efficacy but significantly increased the incidence of side effects, resulting in an overall worse benefit-to-risk assessment for the top dose. Not surprisingly, given the project-specific differences in scope of phase 2 clinical studies, costs and durations for phase 2 are variable, with durations ranging from 12 to 36 months and costs from £6 million to £20 million. During phase 2, the drug synthetic route will ideally have been optimized and "frozen" such that the API used for the long-term toxicity studies and for the phase 3 clinical supplies will have consistent impurity profiles to the API planned for market introduction.

4. Phase 3 development focuses on providing a registration dossier, which provides a clear benefit-to-risk justification for the use of a drug in a defined patient group for a specific clinical intent. The product-label intent needs to be reflected in the phase 3 trial protocols. The commercial intent must be aligned with the hypothesis to be tested in the phase 3 trials. Must the product offer superior efficacy to a marketed competitor product or is the commercial strategy based upon demonstrating noninferiority to the competitor with other product benefits driving the market opportunity? The trial hypothesis will have an important influence on the design of the study and the scale of patient recruitment and hence duration and costs. For chronic therapy drugs, it will be expected that long-term drug exposure will form a key safety component of the dossier with significant numbers of patients (e.g., >500) dosed for 6 to 12 months. Phase 3 typically may take 18 to 40 months to complete. The analysis and report of the vast amount of clinical data needed to create the clinical registration documents may take six months from the end of patient dosing. The cost of phase 3 may be £15 million to over £100 million. The registration dossiers for some projects may exceed 10,000 patients.

5. The registration phase for a project encompasses the period from dossier submission to regulatory agency approval for the drug to be marketed. The review period may be 12 months or more, though faster 6-month reviews may be completed for products given priority review. During the registration phase, the clinical program generally continues to run with additional trials being conducted, which are intended to provide data to support the marketing of the product (phase 3b marketing studies) or studies exploring new indications for the drug.

6. LCM encompasses a broad range of further investments in the product to maximize the commercial revenues. These investments include registration of new indications for the drug, conduct and completion of studies committed to during the registration process (phase 4 commitments), market-driven comparative studies, and new formulations and dose regimens. The scope and scale of LCM investments frequently dwarf the initial registration costs. With a good new product, a pharma company has the opportunity to "raise the hurdle" to future competitors by defining a new standard of care. During LCM trials, the rapidly expanding patient-safety database will become of a size that reveals rare adverse drug effects that may not be detectable at the time of registration approval when potentially only 2000 to 3000 patients may have been studied. LCM investments continue throughout the life of the product until an active disinvestment decision is taken as patent life becomes exhausted (many LCM activities focus on patent-extension strategies). It is difficult to describe "typical" LCM investments. It suffices to say that in some therapeutic areas multiple clinical studies costing in excess of £30 million have been conducted for particular drugs to optimize the market opportunity. The postmarketing trials for several "statins" are an example of heavy investment in large-scale trials to demonstrate mortality benefit due to long-term treatment of atherosclerosis by drugs controlling cholesterol synthesis.

In summary, drug development requires high levels of investment over a long time scale to bring a drug to market and to fully exploit its market potential. The scale of investment increases considerably in later phases. Development projects are risky ventures and substantial investments are at risk, particularly at the late stages of development. The next section examines project attrition.

Project Attrition: Why Most Projects Are Terminated

Very few projects become products. Development costs escalate sharply with each development stage. The later the termination decision, the greater is the investment loss. Project teams and companies often postpone painful termination decisions, thus incurring wasted cost and resources.

The reasons why projects are terminated are worth considering carefully. It is important to separate hard facts from "spin." The hard facts are the number of new medicines licensed for sale in the major markets year after year. They are woefully small in number. In the period from 2001 to 2006, the combined number of new molecular entities and biopharmaceuticals approved by FDA were 29, 24, 27, 36, 20, and 22. In contrast, during the period from 1996 to 2000, the numbers were 56, 45, 37, 39 and 29 (2). Despite the massive advances in science in the past decade, the harsh truth is that fewer new medicines are entering the market. Why?

It is worthwhile stepping back two decades to look again at the debate on project attrition to see if anything of value has been learned. In September 1986, at the 20th Anniversary Meeting of the Society for Drug Research held in London, an important research presentation was made by Walker and Parrish on "Innovation and New Drug Development," which made a serious attempt to define key issues in drug development, including reasons for project attrition. The presentation is as relevant today as it was then, an enduring mirror faced at the industry inviting creative solutions to enhance productivity. The Centre for Medicines Research data, collected from pharmaceutical companies, cited the major categories of data that played the key role in project-termination decisions. This data is illustrated in Figure 1.

In Figure 1, the upper pie diagram displays the whole dataset for a total of 198 projects. The lower pie diagram shows the results for 121 projects, which excluded the anti-infective projects. By comparing the two diagrams, it is evident that pharmacokinetic inadequacy was responsible for terminating nearly all the anti-infective projects and "skews" the picture for other therapeutic areas. Considering the lower diagram for noninfective projects, the major reason given for failure was lack of efficacy. This might reflect a complete lack of efficacy in humans for a novel class of drugs, which showed evidence of efficacy in animal studies. Some pharmaceutical companies set a minimum proportion of their development portfolio as "precedented" in an attempt to reduce the risk. Toxicity is also an important reason to terminate projects. Project teams spend considerable time assessing the impact of toxicology results on their project. The objective of conducting toxicology studies is to define target-organ toxicities and so it should not be a surprise that toxicity findings will be reported to the team. The team will then review the nature and severity of the lesions, the potential to detect and monitor such toxicity in humans, and whether there is an adequate safety margin to the intended human exposure. It is instructive to review the Summary Basis of Approval (SBA) documents (available for review on the FDA Web site) for registered well-known "blockbuster" drugs. Earlier project teams have successfully addressed findings highlighted in animal toxicity studies by conducting preclinical and clinical investigational studies, which have mitigated safety concerns to enable market approval often with initial postmarketing monitoring requirement. The Mevacor SBA is a good case study illustrating intelligent development thinking and response to toxicology findings. Adverse effects in humans may be detected at any stage. In some cases, the first-in-human study may reveal adverse events during the dose escalation such that attainment of the predicted therapeutic dose is not viable. In other cases, it may be late in phase 3 that uncommon serious safety findings emerge when more than 2000 patients have been studied. Pharmacokinetic

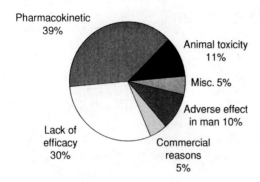

All NCEs (n = 198)

Pharmacokinetic 39%
Animal toxicity 11%
Misc. 5%
Adverse effect in man 10%
Lack of efficacy 30%
Commercial reasons 5%

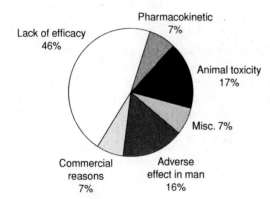

Excluding Anti-Infectives
(n = 121)

Lack of efficacy 46%
Pharmacokinetic 7%
Animal toxicity 17%
Misc. 7%
Commercial reasons 7%
Adverse effect in man 16%

Figure 1   Why do projects fail?

reasons are a significant reason for stopping projects. This could include insufficient bioavailability or excessive variability for an oral drug or perhaps an inappropriate half-life for the drug (too long or too short). Such deficiencies should be detected early in the project thus minimizing wasted investment (3). Commercial reasons to terminate the project could include market reassessment with a conclusion that the chance of an adequate return is too low. Underlying reasons might include pricing and reimbursement issues and inadequate margins on sale (costs of goods, royalty payments to other parties). In addition, the market environment may have changed significantly with the introduction of new and better competitor products.

Table 2 shows the typical failure rate for each phase of development and uses these attrition rates and average phase durations to create a "steady-state" portfolio, which would deliver one new drug per year to successful registration. The table

Table 2 Project Attrition Rates During Development Phases

Phase	Preclinical	1	2	3	NDA
Input	9	7.5	2.5	1.25	1
Output	7.5	2.5	1.25	1	
Elimination	1.5	5	1.25	0.25	
Elimination rate	1/5	2/3	1/2	1/5	
Phase duration	0.9	1	1.5	1.75	
Chance of NDA (%)	11	13	40	80	
Drugs in phase	8.1	7.5	3.75	2.19	

Abbreviation: NDA, new drug application.

shows the input, output, and elimination for each phase. Of nine projects starting preclinical development, only one project will be taken to registration submission. The elimination rate is particularly high in phase 1 and 2 development. The high failure rates in these two phases of development is understandable given the earlier cited causes of project termination. Lack of efficacy, animal toxicity, pharmacokinetic deficiencies, and overt clinical adverse events will generally manifest themselves during phase 1 and 2 and enable the project team to make a sound termination decision. It is very important that nonviable projects are terminated before phase 3 when development investment and organizational resource usage spiral. Table 2 shows a low risk of failure in phase 3 with 80% of projects making it through this phase to registration. Many companies have experienced much higher attrition rates at this stage. This has led to much debate to understand why project teams and senior management seemingly are failing to recognize nonviable projects earlier. Project progression decision making and the decision-making process itself, therefore, are of critical importance to the strategic management of projects (4). Table 2 data can be used to build a steady-state portfolio to get a feel for the size and phase distribution of projects, which would be needed to support a steady flow of products to the market. The base assumptions driving this model are the elimination rate by phase and the duration of each phase. This model predicts that a portfolio of about 22 projects would be required to furnish one new drug application (NDA) per year. Moreover, the distribution of projects would be expected to be heavily stacked at the preclinical and phase 1 stage of development, where 15 of the 22 projects would reside. This type of modeling does give some understanding of why the larger pharmaceutical companies with aspirations for three to four NDAs per year need to have broad pipelines to stand much chance of delivery. In fact, Table 2 likely underestimates the required portfolio because not all projects submitted for registration approval are approved. Perhaps of more concern to the industry is the fact that a significant proportion of projects that are launched never pay back their development investment. This would suggest that companies are setting the bar too low in taking some late-phase projects to the market.

Has the picture of project attrition changed in recent years? Possibly, it has. Kola and Landis (5) cited data for the period from 1991 to 2000 for the top 10 pharma companies for the clinical stages of development. The overall failure rate from phase 1 to approval was 89%. About 60% of drugs made it from phase 1 to phase 2 and only 23% then to phase 3 of which half made it to registration submission. If these attrition rates are compared with those in Table 2, it can be seen that the rate of attrition in phase 2 is higher in the more recent series and most notably phase 3 attrition is very much higher. This is bad news as it indicates that vast resources are being wasted on failed projects as companies fail to spot nonviable projects early enough. It raises the question of whether drug companies really understand drug development decision making. This topic is a major theme of this chapter.

DEFINING THE PROJECT STRATEGY AND PLAN

This section describes how project teams establish a strategy for their project and how they capture and communicate the strategy within the company. "Project nomination" is driven by the discovery organization when a drug candidate has met the criteria approved by the pharma management. There is active involvement from development in the approval process. With approval, the primary responsibility for the project moves from discovery to development. An international project team (IPT) is established and tasked to elaborate an integrated development plan (IDP). The IDP is presented to the development committee to gain its approval for the resources and expenditures needed to progress the project. The project may be a "homegrown" project or an in-licensed project. Companies often have a therapeutic focus so that relevant internal competencies and external advisory panels are in place to guide clinical and marketing strategy. The newly formed IPT has representatives of all the disciplines (Fig. 2). The IPT generally will follow these steps:

- Review of the scientific rationale for the project and the preclinical primary pharmacology results. *"What is the scientific rationale for the project and what benefits do the preclinical studies show?"*
- Development of a clinical strategy defining product benefits to specific patient populations not satisfied by current or pipeline drugs. *"On the basis of the preclinical evidence and an awareness of medical need, which patients will benefit the most from this drug?"*
- Development of a target product profile (TPP) to ensure that the company understands how the intended product will be differentiated from competitor products and what the product labeling will state. *"What specifically is the product that will be prescribed to these patients? What will the product labeling state?"*
- Creation of an integrated project plan that enables the company to understand the scope of the investment, the short-term and long-term

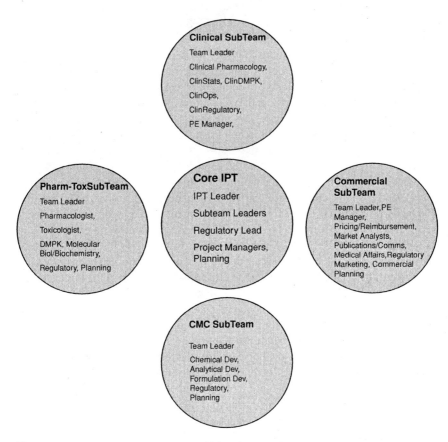

Figure 2 International project team and it's subteams.

objectives of the development plan, and the risks and the potential commercial returns. *"What is the investment needed and why should we invest in this project?"*

By the time a new project is nominated, a lot of discussion will already have taken place about the first two above points but often the TPP is rather embryonic.

The Target Product Profile

The TPP is a critical strategic tool in drug development in defining, for the project team and the broader organization, a clear vision of the product intent. The TPP describes the specification of the product intended to be introduced to the market. It defines the patients who will be prescribed the drug and the indication for use of the drug. It specifies the efficacy performance and the safety profile, the dosing regimen, and how the product is supplied. The target cost of goods will be set and also the planned date of introduction. The TPP is drafted by the whole project team and this exercise ensures that everyone understands the product being "built" and their discipline's contributions to it. Often discussion revolves around "must" and "want" elements of the performance requirements. It is important that the minimum ("must") requirements are defined in the TPP because the project team does need to know where the boundary conditions for project viability lie. Team discussion is facilitated if "must," "want," and "expected" fields are captured in the TPP. The "expected" field is helpful in getting teams to actively review the existing project data against the "must" and "want" fields. Commercially desirable attributes ("wants") should be captured as these may support specific early investment to try to provide a more valuable product, but it is essential that "must" and "want" elements are clearly discriminated. Table 3 shows a format that can be used for the TPP and this example will be discussed in more detail later.

The TPP, in effect, is a contract established at a point in time between the project team and the company. Management approval of the TPP and the budget for the next phase of project activities are conditional upon the project team delivering the agreed TPP. There is scope to "trade off" attributes within a TPP. For example, efficacy may be better than expected and therefore the marketing "must" for a once-daily oral dosing regimen may be relegated to a "want" because the product efficacy will be the key driver for marketing the product against the market "gold standard" comparator. What is not justifiable is a general lowering of TPP target performance simply to allow the horse to clear the fence. The TPP invariably will evolve during development as it reflects not only the findings on the new drug being developed but also the evolution of the competitive landscape in the market, which likely will have changed during the five to six years of development. It is important to carefully reassess and, as appropriate, reset the TPP at each phase progression because internal findings and external market events may have reshaped the product opportunity options.

In the following section, a TPP has been created for a *fictitious* new class of anticoagulant called "Staminex," which is a potent and selective inhibitor of "factor 32a," a protease recently recognized as playing an important regulating role in coagulation and hemostasis.

The discovery team demonstrated that Staminex was effective in a number of preclinical models of thrombosis. Due to its mode of action and its pharmacokinetics, it has the potential as a once-daily drug in several indications, which include short- and long-term prophylaxis indications including the prevention of venous thromboembolism (VTE) in patients undergoing knee surgery, long-term secondary prevention of VTE after standard treatment for an episode of acute VTE, and prevention of stroke and other thromboembolic complications associated with atrial fibrillation. The IPT defined separate TPP for each of the potential indications reviewing the product opportunity, potential differentiation, the label required, the clinical studies needed to secure the label, and the estimated time to market. The major markets for each indication were researched to understand current practices. Product labeling of the gold standard products, deficiencies of existing therapy, and results of clinical trials for drugs in development were assessed. The IPT brought together their assessment of the costs, time, risks, and commercial return for the development of Staminex in the three indications and recommended a sequential registration of indications with market entry being sought for a prevention of VTE in orthopedic surgery patients dosed for 10 days with subsequent filings for long-term prophylaxis claims. Although the commercial value of this short-term indication is less than that of the extended prophylaxis and treatment indications, it enables early market entry with establishment of the brand and expansion of indications as clinical data for long-term prophylaxis become available.

The development of the TPP for the indication "prevention of VTE in patients undergoing knee replacement" will now be described in a greater detail to illustrate some of the practical and strategic issues that typically arise.

In the absence of prophylactic anticoagulation, orthopedic surgery patients are at significant risk of developing VTE. The relative risk is related to age and to the type of surgery. The benefit of prophylaxis is assessed in a composite primary end point that monitors the clinical observations and distinguishes those that signal risk to the patient's well-being and survival. The components of the end point are deep vein thrombosis (DVT) events (defined as being symptomatic and asymptomatic and their location as being distal or proximal), pulmonary embolism, and death. Over several decades, landmark clinical trials and meta-analyses of multiple trials have demonstrated the benefit of prophylaxis in orthopedic surgery. Prophylactic regimens with different pharmacological agents (oral warfarin, subcutaneous low–molecular-weight heparins, and the factor Xa inhibitor, Arixtra) have been shown to improve clinical outcomes. As a result, new drugs attempting to penetrate the market need to differentiate themselves from those market competitors that have already demonstrated impressive efficacy in the level of risk reduction. Thus, while it is known from historical placebo-controlled trials that post–hip surgery total VTE rates may be 40% to 60% in high-risk untreated patients, modern regimens have reduced incidence rates 10-fold in some trials. The consequence is that very large trials will be needed to demonstrate better efficacy than existing approved drugs and to provide regulatory agencies with evidence of superiority. However, market penetration may be driven by product attributes other than efficacy. The marketing team believes this to be the case for Staminex.

Table 3 shows the TPP that the team constructed for the market-entry indication "prevention of VTE in patients undergoing knee surgery." In this indication, clinical practice, driven both by cost and clinical considerations, has seen shorter in-hospital stays for patients undergoing orthopedic surgery. Early mobility and discharge are considered clinically desirable. As a result, a simple oral anticoagulant regimen, which can be continued on discharge, is ideal. There are two gold-standard drugs for this indication. The low–molecular-weight

Table 3 Target Product Profile

Product attribute	Must	Want	Expected	Current market gold standard		Future market gold standard
				Europe, North America	U.S.A.	
Product	Staminex	Staminex	Staminex	LMWH[a] Enoxaparin (Lovenox)	Warfarin	Oral anticoagulants in phase 2/3 (DTs, factor Xa inhibitors, PAR regulators)
Route of administration	Oral	Oral	Oral	Subcutaneous	Oral	Oral
Product form	Tablet or capsule	Tablet	Tablet	Prefilled syringe	Tablet	Tablet or capsule bid and od potentially
Dose regimen	bid	od	od	Europe: 40 mg every 24 hr, initial dose 12 hr presurgery North America: 30 mg every 12 hrs, initial dose 12–24 hrs postsurgery	Not approved for this indication. Consult expert guidelines for use	
Duration of therapy	10-day daily dosing	10-day daily dosing	10-day daily dosing	10–14 days	Guidelines suggest 7–10 days	10 days
Efficacy Primary endpoint Total VTE[b] and all-cause mortality	Noninferior to enoxaparin	Superior to enoxaparin	Superior to enoxaparin based upon primary pharmacology	Total VTE: 26.6% in EXPRESS study Total VTE and all-cause mortality: 37% in REMODEL study	Asymptomatic VTE: 20.7% Proximal VTE: 4.8%	Similar efficacy seen for DTs trialled

Safety/Tolerability

					Dabigatran (DTI)
Bleeding risk Incidence of major and minor bleedings	Noninferior to enoxaparin	Superior to enoxaparin	Superior to enoxaparin from preclinical pharmacology and toxicology results	Major bleeds in about 5% in hip and about 1% for knee surgery trials	Major bleeding in about 3% in hip surgery when INR is 2–3	reported as having similar bleeding risk rate to Lovenox
Adverse safety liabilities	Incidence/severity not limiting to benefit/risk for use in indication	No clinically important safety liabilities	Superior to enoxaparin Predictable PK/PD	Thrombocytopenia, injection sites adverse events (pain, bruising, nodules, and rash)	Skin and muscle necrosis, teratogenicity	Oral dosed drugs without the liability of injection site adverse events
Drug interaction liability	No clinically important ones	None	PK interaction not expected	No PK interaction but dynamic interaction with others hemostatics	Multiple. P450 CYP2C9 highly protein bound	Insufficient data available
Monitoring Need	No	No	No	No	Yes (INR)	No
Renal function	Predictable PK/renal status	No dose adjustment	No dose adjustment	Dose reduction in severe renal impairment <30 mL/min	Lower dose in severe impairment <30 mL/min	Limited data

Abbreviations: LMWH, low–molecular-weight heparin; DTI, direct thrombin inhibitor; PAR, protease activated receptor; bid, twice a day; od, once daily; VTE, venous thromboembolism; INR, international normalized ratio; PK; PD.

heparin enoxaparin (Lovenox), which is given by subcutaneous injection, is approved and marketed for this indication in Europe and North America and is the dominant subcutaneous product for this indication. In the United States, an oral vitamin-K antagonist, warfarin, is recommended by expert guidelines for use in orthopedic surgery to prevent VTE postsurgery but it is not, in fact, an FDA-approved drug for this short-term prophylaxis (it is approved for long-term prophylaxis). Warfarin is an old drug that has limitations as described in the TPP. A new oral drug with a simple regimen and with predictable anticoagulant effect requiring no monitoring would capture this market. New oral drugs with novel modes of action are in phase 2 or 3 evaluation, targeting the same indications as Staminex. Lovenox dose regimens differ in Europe and North America. This makes a global clinical trial program problematic, as companies need to conduct trials for the major markets, comparing with the local gold standard dosed with the approved dose regimen in comparator trials. In the United States, low–molecular-weight heparin and oral warfarin are both recommended (American College of Chest Physicians Guidelines) for VTE prophylaxis in elective hip and knee replacement surgery and in hip fracture surgery. To capture the U.S. warfarin market, it is important to have a Staminex–warfarin comparator trial so as to demonstrate the clinical advantages Staminex has over warfarin. Since warfarin is not formally approved for this indication it may be judged as a "placebo," necessitating that Staminex demonstrates superiority in the study if the study is to be used to gain marketing approval. The clinical trial program that emerges from the clinical, regulatory, and marketing requirements exhibited in the TPP indicate the need to run noninferiority comparator studies against Lovenox in the United States and Europe with the relevant Lovenox regimens and a superiority study against warfarin in the United States if this study is intended as a pivotal efficacy study. The likelihood of achieving superiority would need careful consideration. However, during the development of Staminex, the competitor situation will likely change with the possibility that one or more oral novel anticoagulants currently in late-stage development will be approved. If these are approved, the IPT will need to review again what the gold standard comparator should be with the prospect that a noninferiority phase 3 study could be run against the newly approved competitor oral drug as a pivotal efficacy study. Alternatively, depending on the development schedule of Staminex, it is possible that this study would be conducted during or after the approval of Staminex as a phase 3b or phase 4 study to support marketing objectives.

The Integrated Development Plan

The IDP brings together into one document the business case for investing in a project in the short and the long term. The IDP defines through the TPP the intended product planned to be introduced to the market and when it will be available for sale. The route to market is traced with the description of phases of development activities planned. A project plan defining the schedule of activities and the costs is prepared. The overall development costs are estimated to registration and launch. The commercial return in estimated worldwide sales is projected for a defined period postproduct launch. Net revenues are estimated based on the projected cost of goods. Risk assessment is made for the project and generally a financial calculation will be made of the current value of the project for the purpose of judging relative attractiveness of investment in the project in comparison with other projects in the company portfolio (refer to chap. 2 for further discussion).

The IDP can easily become a heavy treatise if the process for its creation is poorly managed. Many companies have templates to help teams prepare an IDP. The audience for the IDP is the development committee, functional heads in discovery, development, and marketing and the IPT itself. The IDP will be revised at each key stage in development. Typically, the initial plan while tracing the route to market will also set short-term objectives and define decision criteria to move to the next development stage. Sometimes, the preclinical data will define an expectation for demonstration of proof of concept in an early clinical study, which can be used to decide whether further investment is justified. A balance needs to be struck between the need to trace the route to market for an early plan, which strategically is important, while avoiding wasteful and excessive detailed planning of later-phase activities, which likely will never be undertaken. Experienced development companies can draw from historic or "generic plans" to make reasonable estimates of costs and times for later-phase studies (see chap. 10). Decision-making committees, which are regularly reviewing a number of projects, value a concise, focused IDP that makes an honest assessment of challenges and opportunities and clearly highlights the key assumptions upon which the project viability rests. An example of the content of an IDP is summarized in Table 4. This plan was for a project in phase 1 for which the IPT wanted approval of resources and funds to take the project to registration. While not prescriptive, it is generally possible to create an IDP of 35 to 40 pages providing adequate information to an oversight committee to make an informed decision. In bigger companies, more detailed plans exist within the functions. It is worth highlighting that project investment decisions made by the oversight committee are driven in part by the IDP, in part by the presentation to the committee, and in part by informal briefings between team members, line function managers, and committee members.

Project Viability and Investment Decisions

Since most projects fail it is not surprising that pharma companies have tried to get smarter at spotting nonviable projects. It is instructive to consider this from two perspectives. Firstly, from the perspective of the company owning the asset. Secondly, from the perspective of an external party considering acquiring the asset. External parties will subject a project to "due diligence" evaluation. In theory, pharma companies should apply the same due-diligence rigor and scrutiny to decide whether internal projects merit progression to the next stage of

Table 4   The Integrated Development Plan

Plan section	Pages	Content	Comment
Executive summary	4	The approval sought (scope of activities, funds, and resources) Development strategy Key risks/risk management Go/no-go checkpoint and criteria High level Gantt chart	A template often used so that the oversight committee has consistent "view" of the projects being presented
Target product profile(s)	2	Refer to Table 3	The detail increases during development phases
Business strategy	5	Market definition Marketing assumptions Pharmacoeconomics strategy	Current and future market structure and constraints to access
Clinical strategy	5	Clinical strategy Clinical studies tabulation Clinical Gantt chart Clinical issues/issue management	High level extract from a functional clinical plan
Regulatory strategy	3	Regulatory strategy Regulatory plan Regulatory risks/risk management	Defines regulatory strategy/plans for the major markets
Technical strategy CMC	3	Drug substance plan Drug product plan Analytics plan Key issues/issue management	The manufacturing strategy for sourcing and supply detailed in functional plans
Scientific summary	4	Scientific rationale Preclinical plan ADME plan Key issues/issue management	High-level status summary and forward activity plan
Development costs	2	Estimated costs by stage Estimated costs by activity type	Standardized analyses for portfolio
Financial analysis	4	5th-yr revenues Financial assessment of project	Standardized analyses for portfolio

Abbreviations: CMC, chemistry, manufacturing and controls; ADME, absorption, distribution, metabolism, excretion.

development. Interestingly, there is evidence that licensed projects are more likely to be successfully developed to market (6), justifying the belief that in the land of "not invented here" the barrier is held higher for licensed products thereby selecting a higher proportion of thoroughbreds.

Project termination may result from an IPT recommendation because of "single issues" that are encountered, such as unacceptable toxicity in animals or in clinical trials. In addition, the IPT may judge that a combination of factors mean that a TPP will not likely be met and recommend termination. Terminations may also happen because an oversight committee reviewing a project IDP concludes that the risk or return is unacceptable. This assessment may be influenced by portfolio considerations because it would be better if resources were diverted to stronger projects.

When a pharma company considers for licensing a drug, a due-diligence team of functional experts is sent to the licensing company to review the data and discuss it with their experts. If they are well organized, they focus intently on the "big 5" questions to the licensing company:

1. Do they "own" the drug?
2. Do they have a viable drug-product form?
3. Is their drug "fit for use" for its planned clinical indication(s)?
4. Is there a real market opportunity for their drug?
5. Can we get a worthwhile return on the investment in the drug?

These questions need to be considered with the same intensity internally at each stage of drug development. A formal review of the big 5 is fully justified to counter inevitable project "drift" and all five questions have to be positively answered. The information to answer the questions at a phase-transition review is often insufficient, particularly in the earlier stages of development. However, project "signatures" often do emerge quite early and signal likely nonviability. The cross-functional groups that work together to assess these big 5 questions generally, if they are experienced, speak a common language and bring a powerful combined expertise to assess viability. For example, for question 3, a review of "benefit to risk" brings together pharmacologists, toxicologists, pharmacokineticists, clinical pharmacologists, clinicians, and often statisticians. There is a shared understanding of data limitations, signal to noise, relative drug exposure, and frailty of extrapolation that enables these professionals reach a balanced conclusion regarding the benefit-to-risk assessment at that point in development. The same common understanding and strength in review is there when the chemistry, manufacturing and controls (CMC) disciplines get together to consider product viability from chemical, analytical, and formulation perspectives. These functions or rather "combined functional groups" along with the relevant expertise to review the big 5 questions can help a company to set robust and relevant hurdles at phase-transition reviews.

The other "telescope view" is an integrated view spanning all disciplines that comes together most clearly within the full project team. Projects may be nonviable because of a single issue. However, the interlinking features of the project often fatally compromise project viability. For example, low bioavailability + complex chemical synthesis + royalty obligation + competitive product pricing may prevent an adequate margin on sales for the new drug. The viability of a project must therefore be critically evaluated by reassessing whether the TPP will likely be achieved in light of recent development findings and fresh assessment of the competitive product environment at the time of product launch.

Table 5 shows one approach to structuring the phase-transition review process. The review ideally should bring together the strength of the project team's intimate knowledge and understanding of the project that comes from their day-to-day project involvement. In addition, functional review and endorsement of the key phase-transition summaries add real value to the assessment enabling senior management to make informed decisions. During the review process, the involvement of relevant external experts is of great value as part of the functional review to avoid a company "tunnel vision" perspective. The project team should prepare the TPP "scoreboard" as described above for function and senior management review. In addition, concise summary documents should be prepared for the big 5 questions. These questions naturally would be reviewed by the patents function ("product ownership is secure"), the CMC function ["product form(s) are viable"], a benefit-to-risk assessment group involving preclinical and clinical expertise ("product is fit for use"), and marketing ("product has real market opportunity"). The project management staff would prepare with the project team a detailed costed and scheduled development plan for the next phase (with lighter definitions of subsequent project studies). The project team then would integrate the proposal to senior management as an investment recommendation including discussion on the potential market return, the estimated overall development costs to market introduction for a defined indication, next-phase costs, and the project risk assessment addressing the chance of delivering the TPP. Generally, a risk-adjusted return on investment analysis will be done. Inevitably, the precision of information at the early stage of development is more limited and the product is many years from market. The review process for early-phase projects can be sensibly adapted to avoid an unrealistic expectation of precision.

DEVELOPMENT STRATEGIES TO OPTIMIZE A PRODUCT

The remainder of this chapter will discuss development strategies in some key project areas. The fields selected are the ones that invariably have a major impact on the success or failure of the project.

Product Ownership Strategy

Ownership of the asset is vital to recouping the huge cost to discover, develop, and market a new drug. The cost of making the drug product may be only 5% to 10% of the market price and generic companies carefully track the expiries of patents

Table 5 Phase-Transition Review

	Preclinical [leading to phase-transition decision (PT-1)]	Phase 1 [leading to phase-transition decision (PT-2)]	Phase 2 [leading to phase-transition decision (PT-3)]	Phase 3 [leading to registration decision (PT-R)]	Registration [leading to market-entry decision (PT-M)]	Life cycle management (Repeated cycles of investment decisions to exploit the asset)
Project viability assessment						
Product ownership is secure	Patents review PT-1 Preclinical studies for new indications	Patents review PT-2 Initiation of INN and trademarks	Patents review PT-3 API process patents Formulation patents	Patents review PT-R	Patents review PT-M	Patents review LCM License rights secure IP for in-licensed formulation technology
Product forms are viable	API/product review PT-1	API/product review PT-2	API/product review PT-3	API/product review PT-R	API/product review PT-M	API/product review LCM
Product is "fit for use" (benefit/risk)	Scientific/clinical review PT-1 Advisory board	Clinical review PT-2 Advisory board Regulatory exchange PT-2	Clinical review PT-3 Advisory board Regulatory exchange PT-3	Clinical review PT-R Advisory board Regulatory exchange PT-3	Clinical/medical marketing review PT-M Advisory board	Clinical/medical marketing review LCM Advisory board
Product has real market opportunity	Marketing review PT-1 PE step1 Key markets-1	Marketing review PT-2 PE step 2 Key markets-2	Marketing review PT-3 PE step 3 Key markets-3	Marketing review PT-R PE step R Key markets-R	Marketing review PT-M PE step M Key markets-M	Marketing review PT-M LCM PE LCM Central-funded LCM Local-funded LCM
Further investment is justified	TPP at PT-1 Development plan PT-1 Risk assessment Role analysis	TPP at PT-2 Development plan PT-1 Risk evaluation Role analysis	TPP at PT-3 Development plan PT-2 Risk evaluation Role analysis	TPP at PT-R Development plan PT-3 Risk evaluation Role analysis	TPP at PT-M Development plan PT-M Risk evaluation Role analysis	TPP LCM indications Development plans LCM Risk evaluation Role analysis

Abbreviations: PT, phase transition; INN, international non-proprietary names; API, active pharmaceutical ingredient; PE, pharmacoeconomics; TPP, target product profile.

for profitable drugs and are very quick to introduce a generic replacement. Within months, the originator typically will lose the major market share and may indeed decide to terminate the product line soon after. It is the exclusivity to make and sell the product that allows pharmaceutical companies the chance to recover their investments. It is important that the project team and the broader organization continue to explore ways to protect a product for as long as possible from a generic attack. Product protection can be achieved under a variety of mechanisms. These include patents, technical know-how, regulatory exclusivity, trademarks, and design. A variety of patents can be filed and granted that may enable the product to enjoy market exclusivity many years beyond the expiry of the initial composition-of-matter patent granted for the API. Since it often takes a number of years after launch for a new drug to achieve the target market penetration and revenue return, gaining additional years or months of market exclusivity is highly valuable. The project team therefore needs to carefully review the many unexpected and novel findings that typically occur in the discovery and development of a new drug and exploit these opportunities to buttress, broaden, and extend intellectual property rights to the asset. These activities really lie at the heart of the drug development process because product ownership must be made secure for an extended period of marketing. Moreover, while the legal expertise and advice will be available to the project team it is a core responsibility of the team members to be constantly seeking new opportunities. This section in its concision will considerably simplify many aspects of a fairly complex process (7).

For the developer of a new drug, market exclusivity can be gained for a defined period within a particular territory by the grant of a patent. In exchange for this period of exclusivity, the patent holder discloses the nature of the invention such that others within the field would also be able to apply the invention. The patent system, thereby, was intended to benefit the society in spreading the application of new practices, which otherwise would have remained as trade secrets with the inventor. In essence, the patent system can be viewed as a catalyst for innovation in industrial society by ensuring knowledge is shared but also recompensing the inventor. Three key requirements must be met to secure a patent. Firstly, the invention must be novel. Secondly, it must involve an inventive step. Thirdly, it must be capable of industrial application.

Early patent systems evolved during the fifteenth century in England, the Republic of Venice, Germany, France, and the Netherlands; in 1788, powers to grant patents were conferred to the Congress under the Constitution of the United States. Two important differences emerged in the patent process in the United States. Firstly, the inventor must also apply for the patent, whereas elsewhere the application can be assigned to an employer. Secondly, the patent is granted to the person who made the invention rather than the first person to file for it. The grant of a patent will depend on the demonstration of novelty, practical usefulness, and lack of obviousness.

Patents can be filed and granted for the API itself in a composition-of-matter patent, patents for the process of manufacture, patents for formulations

Table 6 Product Ownership

Product ownership rights	Development stage	Comments
Composition-of-matter patent for API and related series of compounds	Typically filed while in discovery when an adequate structure–activity relationship has been defined	Broad claims filed often narrowed in the review process. Grant of patent may take 2–5 yrs during which time IP dominance by other parties may be revealed
API crystal form	In early development, during API synthesis optimization, new crystal forms with unexpected physicochemical advantage may be discovered	Example: GlaxoSmithKline's defense of its polymorph type II of the active ingredient in Zantac against competitors after the patent on polymorph type I had expired
API new salt	Advantages can derive from selection of the right salt form and in early development, switches in salt form are sometimes made	The initial salt selected for development may show poor stability and be replaced with a new salt form providing valuable additional patent cover
New formulation	Often developed for postmarketing life cycle product optimization	Example: controlled release tablet enabling once-a-day dosing
New indication	Novel findings from preclinical or clinical studies at any development stage may reveal clinical utility in new indications	Thalidomide was developed for morning sickness in pregnant women. Later discovered antiangiogenic and immunomodulatory efficacy resulted in its development for treatment of leprosy and lead to patenting
New synthetic processes	Improvements in the synthesis of the API will continue to be sought. The market-entry process is often nonoptimized	Reduction in cost of API drives investment in process optimization and offers new patent opportunities, e.g., switch from costly natural product to fully synthetic product
Patent term extension	IND through the regulatory approval process	An "early" IND potentially may maximize the term extension
Regulatory exclusivity	At product approval Grants the sponsor a period of data exclusivity barring generics companies from using the sponsor's NCE data for an approval	Sponsor needs to avoid data "seepage" Throughout development technical data and information should not be disclosed other than in fulfilling statutory obligations

Abbreviations: IP, intellectual property; API, active pharmaceutical ingredient; IND, investigational new drug; NCE, new chemical entity.

of the drug, and patents for new uses (indications) of the drug (Table 6). During the drug development, the project team will discuss unexpected findings that offer new patenting opportunities. Beyond the discovery of the novel API itself, these might include the discovery of new crystalline and salt forms of advantage. The synthetic process for the API may provide opportunities to patent key steps in which the invention can be demonstrated. The strength of the intellectual property ownership is often described in terms of a web of patents or a "patent thicket" in which the strength of protection resides not in any single granted patent but rather by the strength of the web of patents that prevent other companies from entering the market.

Patent filing should continue through the lifespan of the project until the viable opportunities are truly exhausted. While the initial composition-of-matter patents may have long expired, protection may continue for many years under the formulation and new indication patents and significant manufacturing cost advantage may still be with the originator as a result of adroit process patents.

Patents typically provide the strongest protection of product ownership from generic competitors threatening to create a commodity market. However, product know-how and regulatory exclusivity are also strong elements in maintaining product exclusivity. A vast amount of product information and knowledge is generated during development, which is included in the submission to gain regulatory agency approval to market the new drug. It is important that a company retains and keeps secret such information internally and does not disclose it inadvertently in publications.

In the United States, protection of product exclusivity can be maximized against generic competition by securing the full benefits offered to sponsors by U.S. legislation. Firstly, the patent term extension is provided as a result of the recognition by Congress of the erosion of patent term by the duration of development and regulatory approval of new drugs. In essence, the patent term extension is based upon the duration from the investigational new drug (IND) opening to NDA filing and the duration of the review. (50% IND to NDA, 100% review) with certain limitations (no extension for >5 years, extended patent term should not be >14 years). In addition, regulatory exclusivity provisions can protect the sponsor of the new chemical entity (NCE). The sponsor is entitled to a five-year exclusivity period that bars the submission of a generic drug application that contains that NCE. In practice, generic approvals are generally obtained at least seven years post–NCE approvals as a result of patent challenges and the approval process.

Other "product ownership" elements should not be discounted particularly when considered in the overall context of multiple patent expiries. Trademarks and dosage form design protection are important when key patents preventing generic entry are in place but experience has shown that in reality, once generic competitors enter the market, these elements offer limited protection from rapid sales erosion.

It is important to formally review product ownership and patent strategy at each phase transition to check that the level of security justifies further investment and to challenge project teams to ensure all patenting opportunities are being vigorously exploited. A formal phase-transition "checkpoint" on product ownership is particularly important because in early discovery and development phases it may not be clear whether the patents filed will be granted or whether the scope of the patent may be severely restricted. In addition, the awareness of the competitor patent landscape will evolve during development revealing perhaps that another company holds dominating intellectual property rights impinging upon one of the patents being sought for the product. In such cases, it may be possible to negotiate grant of a license, which may be attractive if the other party has no real product development intent.

Clinical Strategy

Clinical development is circumscribed by reasonably well-established international guidelines that provide clinical teams a basis to trace a clinical development path to registration and launch for a chosen indication. Trial design, conduct, data analysis, and reporting follow defined procedures. The heart of clinical strategy is really about recognizing the clinical potential of a novel drug and how best to demonstrate it. Strong scientific contacts will usually have been established by the discovery group with leading scientists in a particular therapeutic area. With the progression of a project into formal development it is important to establish a clinical advisory group drawn from leading centers of excellence to ensure that clinical strategy decisions are based on a real understanding of patient needs and the evolving treatment options. For novel "first-in-class" drugs, discussion of the in vitro and in vivo preclinical data with the clinical advisory group is useful and often results in helpful suggestions for additional preclinical studies. Most drugs brought to market are not first in class. Valuable lessons are to be learnt from the track history of other "same-in-class" agents, which may influence the design of clinical protocols and/or give valuable operational insights to patient recruitment. In many therapeutic areas, a relatively small number of key opinion leaders have established for themselves an important role in the development of new drugs and potentially can help drug companies define a good development strategy. Some of these individuals will have written or contributed to clinical practice guidelines. They will often have been consulted by regulatory agencies in the benefit-to-risk assessment for a new drug. Building a clinical advisory panel with the right individuals is therefore a key early step. Getting the right balance of representation on the clinical advisory panel is important. The clinical therapeutic area leader will generally know the "environment" and know who are the "popes," who are the upcoming investigators with the drive, intellect, and enthusiasm, and which are the key centers of excellence that need to be involved. They will also know the "all mouth and no action" investigators and the therapeutic area politics and antagonisms. Companies generally try to build an advisory group that brings an international perspective recognizing that treatment paradigms still may differ in major territories.

Having established the clinical advisory group it is very important to get the most value from it by well-structured meetings with clearly defined objectives. The members of the advisory group are invariably very busy individuals who have only limited and intermittent exposure to the project. Concise briefing materials (e.g., clinical study listing, clinical study synopses, next studies, and draft protocol) need to be circulated prior to the meeting together with a list of specific questions the advisory group will be asked to comment on. The agenda needs to be actively managed to ensure that the meeting does not drift into "comfort zone" exchanges offering no direction to development strategy. While time must be given to discuss the background science and its likely clinical relevance, there is also a need to get on to the specifics of best indications, best end points to be studied, trial decision criteria, and the practicalities of trial recruitment. The meeting must be accurately minuted, which includes noting the sometimes discrepant views of the experts on specific issues and the advisory group should get timely copy of the minutes and the chance to add or revise. If well run, the clinical advisory group meeting adds great value to the clinical strategy. The advisory group meetings are scheduled to enable the feedback to be incorporated into finalized trial design for the next phase of development. By establishing the advisory group early in the life of the project, the participants will have already had a chance to become familiar with the background science and a strong working relationship will have been established. For first-in-class drugs, the advice of the experts will be of particular value in identifying possible "proof of concept" studies that could, in reasonable-sized clinical study, provide initial evidence of drug activity that might encourage investment in potentially much larger and expensive trials supporting product registration.

Regulatory Strategy

The development program ultimately seeks to successfully gain marketing approval for the new drug in the major territories around the world with product labeling that enables competitive marketing and a strong commercial return. Regulatory agencies focus on two of the big 5 questions in the product approval process. "Is the product 'fit for use'?" means "Is there adequate evidence that a defined patient group will have an overall benefit from taking the drug as prescribed?" "Is there a 'viable' drug product?" means "Can the sponsor demonstrate adequate control on the manufacturing processes for the drug substance and drug product such that a defined specification is maintained for the shelf life of the product when appropriately stored?" Regulatory agencies were criticized in the past for being bureaucratic and slowing the introduction of valuable new medicines to patients. In more recent times there is clear evidence both from the greater number of rapid approvals and the introduction of a variety of initiatives to harmonize international regulatory requirements that regulatory agencies want to work productively and cooperatively with sponsor companies. To this end, it makes sense to meet with regulatory agencies during the development to gain their concurrence with the proposed strategy and the scope and design of proposed studies. Good preparation is needed for regulatory exchange meetings. A concise briefing documentation and a list of specific questions from the sponsor need to be sent prior to the meeting. It is important to have experienced team members covering the disciplines to be discussed. Backup strategies need thinking through where contentious issues are to be discussed. External experts with therapeutic area expertise can be helpful. For smaller companies, the advice of regulatory consultants with recent experience working within the major agencies can be valuable in recognizing the likely points of contention.

The first significant regulatory "approval" needed is to initiate clinical trials generally in volunteers. Ethics committee approval is granted based on the package of preclinical studies and the CMC package, which will include the product specification and short-term stability covering the planned trial. In the United States, an investigational new drug application is filed to support the clinical trial. The opening of the IND allows the sponsor to progress to clinical trial initiation following institutional ethical committee review. A broadly similar procedure operates in Europe under the clinical trial directive. Generally, sponsor companies try to hold regulatory agency exchange meetings with both the U.S. and European Union regulatory agencies to a similar schedule to try to integrate feedback from both into the final protocols. If the clinical development program is initiated in Europe, companies also generally try to file an IND early in the clinical program to recognize and resolve issues before significant development investment decisions are taken. The end of phase 2 meeting is the key regulatory exchange meeting in gaining concurrence to the proposed registration program. The clinical end points and the statistical plan are important topics discussed, as is the evidence from phase 2 that a dose response for the drug has been defined. The project team will have developed the core data sheet and product-labeling intent, which will be aligned with the commercially endorsed TPP. The CMC data and further manufacturing plans will be shared with the regulatory agencies. Regulatory agencies will look for any changes in the API and product purity and impurity profile, which might indicate that the product tested in the pivotal clinical trials differs from that to be introduced into the market. Sponsor companies will be keen to "freeze" the API synthesis and to supply this drug substance to the phase 3 clinical studies, the long-term toxicology studies, the representative scale-up manufacturing batches, and the market-entry supplies.

Companies can benefit from review of the approval of other drugs since FDA's SBA documentation is open to public scrutiny. While commercially sensitive sections of the NDA submission may be redacted, the core elements of the clinical data are open for review together with the assessment reports of the FDA reviewers. Careful review of the SBA of competitor drugs can give valuable insights in the design of a clinical program. There are a number of opportunities that companies may want to explore for particular drug development programs. For development projects offering evident advance in treatment benefit, it is possible to apply for priority review. This provides for a potentially faster review process, which in 2003 resulted in FDA review times of less than seven months for priority new molecular entities. For drugs that are being developed for smaller patient populations, it is possible to apply for orphan drug designation in the United States if the number of patients is less than 200,000. If orphan drug designation is granted, there are advantages to the sponsor which include no payment for the approval review, grants, and potential tax breaks set against developments, all of which are intended to encourage companies to develop medicines for rarer diseases. The U.S. government, recognizing that the development and review times for new medicines have eroded the period of patent exclusivity, introduced legislation, which allowed companies to seek extended exclusivity under the provision of "regulatory exclusivity." The Waxman–Hatch legislation allows companies to claim for an extension of exclusivity.

Commercial and Pharmacoeconomics Strategy

Increasing healthcare costs have stimulated governments and healthcare providers to challenge whether the cost of new drugs can be justified. Decision makers need to be convinced that the price of a new drug is reasonable for the benefit the drug brings to patient care. The adoption of a new drug into reimbursement schemes can make or break its commercial success. To achieve this, a pharmacoeconomic strategy and plan must be established early in development—it is not a "tag on" activity that starts in phase 3. The project team itself must recognize the importance of this work and give it the time and support it deserves.

There are a number of groups who influence whether a new drug will be prescribed (Fig. 3). This goes beyond the "technical" benefit-to-risk assessment of the regulatory agency. Put simply, a new drug may be technically "better" than an old drug but if it costs 10 times more than old drug, should it be prescribed? The decision of whether the cost of a new drug can be prescribed with reimbursement is taken by different bodies in different countries. In the United Kingdom, the National Institute of Clinical Excellence recommends whether a new drug should be adopted for use within the U.K. health system. In the United States, a variety of managed healthcare schemes are in operation, which will decide whether a new drug is eligible for reimbursement. It is therefore critical that there is a well-thought strategy to ensure that an economic dossier is built during development that demonstrates the full economic value that the new drug brings in the real world clinical setting. An integrated health economics strategy provides data when needed to the relevant customer. In early development, a pharmacoeconomic strategy can be developed with modeling based on epidemiological studies and surveys to define the way disease management is practiced in the major countries. This will help to focus clinical development strategy and to identify the most important data to demonstrate product value in use. This type of study can be

Strategic Project Management at the Project Level

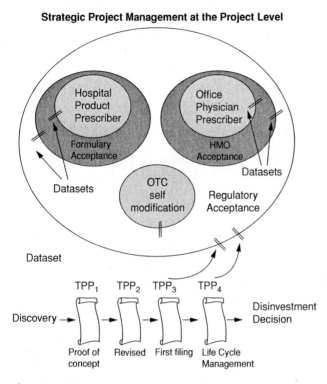

Figure 3   TPP and data for decision makers.

undertaken in phase 1 (or indeed earlier as support to the discovery function's disease area focus) Early development studies should be performed to further define current practices of disease management. This should address the currents options of treating disease and the real world direct and indirect costs and benefits of such interventions. This work provides a basis for assessing the differential impact of intervention with a new drug. Therefore, this type of study should be conducted early in development so that its findings are available in time to influence the protocol design of the phase 3 pivotal trials.

The phase 3 pivotal studies provide an important opportunity to collect important data that can help demonstrate cost effectiveness. The limited scale of such trials, the homogenous nature of patients studied, and the protocol limitations do not make such studies typical of subsequent product use. The collection of data for pharmacoeconomic purposes in such trials is described as a piggyback strategy because the primary driver for such studies is to achieve regulatory approval. The pharmacoeconomics of a new drug are more realistically studied in phase 3b trials conducted after filing and in the post–marketing approval setting in which large patient databases can be assessed to determine short- and long-term benefits, liabilities, and costs. Increasingly continued investment in pharmacoeconomic studies postlaunch will be needed to support a product in the market by generating the data, which break through barriers to prescription.

Speed-to-Market Strategy

Pharma companies have spent a lot of time analyzing ways of reducing time to market through process improvement projects (see chap. 10 for further discussion). Such initiatives are valuable if they bring together line functions and project teams to a better understanding of the drug development process. Generic development plans have been developed for acute and chronic therapies which enable the estimation of "irreducible" development times based upon cycle times for "standard" activities. These generic plans can be useful to "sanity check" schedules built by project teams. Chapter 3 elaborates on project planning in more detail. There is some evidence that big pharma companies have reaped some reward from improving their drug development process. Median development times can be seen to have progressively reduced over the period 1992 to 2001 as reported by Keyhani and colleagues in 2004 (8).

The author led a joint Roche–Gilead development team that took Tamiflu, the "bird flu drug," from phase 1 to a successful registration filing in just over two years. Several factors enabled this rapid development. Firstly, a clear determination by the senior management of both companies that oral Tamiflu be brought to market as close as possible after the launch of the competitor inhaled–flu-antiviral, Relenza, which entered development more than three years earlier. The development of Relenza was likely helpful in spotting development pitfalls. In the United States, the recognition of the health risk posed by pandemic flu created a regulatory environment supportive to the early introduction of new antiflu drugs. The seasonal nature of flu, the short duration of the season (6–8 weeks), and the uncertainty of where it would strike galvanized the clinical operations groups to put in place smart flu detection and rapid recruitment strategies turning a considerable challenge into an opportunity that was successfully exploited. The remarkable pace of the clinical program potentially might have put the manufacturing schedule on the critical path. In fact, the timelines for clinical and CMC activities were planned so that key reports from both areas were available at the designated submission date. Tamiflu was launched in the U.S. market in the same winter season (1999/2000) as Relenza, sidelining the inhaled product.

A number of features of the Tamiflu development are relevant to development strategy. Because Tamiflu is an antiviral, it was possible to get guiding data on its clinical dose response early in a phase 1 flu challenge study. This helped decisions regarding doses to be given to patients. A combined phase 2 and 3 was conducted rather than a traditional phase 2 followed by a phase 3 trial. A significant amount of clinical data and nonclinical data was submitted during the review process. All these factors played a part in shortening the development time enabling a rapid introduction of Tamiflu into the market.

While several planning strategies were successful in achieving rapid market entry for Tamiflu, a cautionary note is appropriate. Attempts to truncate development time often carry risk and may indeed prove counterproductive. In addition, combining phase 2 and phase 3 may look appealing from a scheduling perspective, but the sponsor may be committing to a very expensive clinical program before the efficacy and safety dose–response relationship has been adequately characterized.

There is common ground between regulatory agencies and the industry in the need to bring clinically valuable drugs more quickly to market. The FDA's critical path initiative "Challenge and Opportunity on the Critical Path to New Medicinal Products" is one example. Good project management strategy and a preparedness to be open with regulatory agencies on objectives may enable the sponsor and the regulator to work together more effectively to societal benefit.

ENVOI

This chapter has described how good development strategies can be set for development projects. The phases of drug development were first outlined together with the scale of the costs and time at each phase. Then the risky nature of development was discussed and the reasons why projects fail cited. The impact of the project failure rate was considered from a portfolio perspective. The need for a rigorous decision making process to kill weak projects and minimize wasted investment was emphasized. This led into a discussion of how project viability should be assessed. The critical importance of both the due-diligence big 5 questions and the TPP in decision making was highlighted. A process for phase-transition review was recommended. The elements of the TPP were outlined and a TPP case study for a fictitious new oral antithrombotic drug was used to exemplify it. The IPT was described, as was the process, whereby the TPP and the integrated project plan were elaborated. In the final section, recommendations were made on project strategy in some critical areas, which the project team must address. These included strategies to optimize proprietary rights, clinical and regulatory strategy, commercial and pharmacoeconomic strategy, and speed to market strategy.

Drug development is an extraordinary working environment. It is populated with exceptionally talented people from the many disciplines that contribute to new medicines. Managing drug development effectively matters. It makes the difference between success and failure for both individual projects and companies. A sound understanding of drug development and of the strategies that can foster success is therefore important.

REFERENCES

1. Guidelines for Phase 1 Clinical Trials. 2007 Published by the Association of the British Pharmaceutical Industry. www.abpi.org.uk/publications/pdfs/phase1 guidelines.pdf.

2. Owens J. 2006 Drug approvals; finding the niche. Nat Rev Drug Discov 2007; 6:99–101.
3. Wang J, Urban L. The impact of early ADME profiling on drug discovery and development strategy. Drug Discov World (Fall 2004); 15:73–86.
4. Kennedy T. Managing the drug discovery/development interface. Drug Discov Today. 1997; 2(Suppl 10):436–444.
5. Kola I, Landis J. Can the pharmaceutical industry reduce attrition rates? Nat Rev Drug Discov 2004; 3:711–716.
6. Benjamin G, Lumley C. Industry success rates 2003 including trends in success rates. CMR reports No 03-202 R. CMR International, U.K., 2003.
7. Grubb P. Patents for Chemicals, Pharmaceuticals and Biotechnology. Oxford University Press, U.K., 2004.
8. Keyhani S, Diener-West M, Powe N. Are development times for pharmaceuticals increasing or decreasing? Health Aff 2006; 25(Suppl 2):461–468.

2

Strategic Project Management at the Portfolio Level

Kevin Bilyard
Nine-TZ Healthcare Ventures, Wilmslow, Cheshire, U.K.

Des Markland
Decanalysis Ltd., Congelton, Cheshire, U.K.

WHAT ARE THE AIMS OF PORTFOLIO MANAGEMENT?

Introduction

It is worth reflecting on some historical features of the pharmaceutical industry. The predecessors of several of today's major players were companies operating in related fields, typically industrial chemicals, retail healthcare, or foods. While there may have been some technical synergies, the market for prescription pharmaceuticals has developed in a completely different way to the markets for products from the original core businesses, and few would dispute that the pharmaceuticals industry has, in general, offered a greater value to shareholders. However, without the sponsorship, often over periods of decades, of these less-glamorous parent companies, many of the names that we today associate exclusively with pharmaceuticals would not exist, let alone be among some of the most highly valued global businesses.

In the period from 1960 to 1980, both extremes were exemplified—the transformational potential of successful products (antibiotics, beta blockers, H_2 antagonists, etc.) and the destructive consequences of an unsuccessful product (thalidomide). This served to fuel the debate as to whether focusing on higher value pharmaceuticals compared to, for example, commodity chemicals was the way to go. Glaxo is an example of a company that essentially rebuilt its business around pharmaceuticals with considerable success and today many people would be unaware of its original interests in baby food and other nonpharmaceutical products. Some organizations remained more circumspect, perhaps because they were still waiting for the elusive "blockbuster" product and spending a lot in getting there. These businesses, typified by the chemical conglomerates such as ICI in the United Kingdom and Bayer or Hoechst in Germany seemed to take the view that the cash generated by other business units was essential to fund the highly R&D-intensive pharmaceutical operations. It was only when a profitable pharmaceutical product emerged, inspiring rapid growth, that arguments began to surface about the pharmaceutical business units being constrained by policies and practices designed for different customers and markets. The counterargument about the logic of keeping everything together to mitigate risk and "smoothen" the cyclical profile of those business units that are more susceptible to general economic trends prevailed for a while. However, the dominant trend was to create dedicated, independent pharmaceutical companies. The most successful of these companies soon became cash rich but the search for the next big product proved challenging and costly in many cases. The inefficiency of the R&D process became evident and new regulations introduced to promote safety resulted in further escalation of costs and increased timescales. Increasing competition with many similar products reaching the market meant significantly higher sales and marketing costs. The relative simplicity of the company with a dominant product in the market and a modest, easily absorbed R&D operation was certainly a thing of the past. Larger portfolios with resources constrained by internal economic factors created an urgent need for more revenue-generating products to feed the larger cost base. Astute in-licensing of late-stage products provided some relief for those companies able to secure the deals, but only temporarily. Even during the 1980s, consolidation through merger or acquisition was predicted to be the only option for many companies with the vision that the industry would be dominated by a relatively small number of mega-companies by the turn of the century. In general, this prediction became a reality but it does not seem to have solved the fundamental problem of R&D productivity. Improving the effectiveness and efficiency of the R&D process is an increasingly important objective for most companies. Portfolio management, the subject of this chapter, is aligned with effectiveness—picking the winners, as some would say—whereas project management is more about efficiency or ensuring that the selected products are developed economically. So, what does portfolio management seek to do when applied correctly? Correctly applied portfolio management

- provides a structure for decision-making when multiple projects are competing for common, limited resources.
- allows common methods to be used for comparing the attractiveness of projects.
- creates a group of projects that has the potential to meet the overall objectives of the business.
- minimizes investment in projects that are judged unlikely to achieve the technical profile required for commercial success.
- does all of the above on a dynamic basis.

The challenges are many and include

- reluctance to make decisions resulting in hedging tactics that try to keep everything going.
- inability to agree on methods of evaluation coupled with an "art more than science" mentality.
- insufficient clarity or definition of what the business is trying to achieve and therefore no means of grouping projects accordingly.
- the sentiment that most successes are unpredictable and occur in spite of target profiles and contrary commercial opinion.
- a feeling that, however sophisticated, portfolio management can only be a simplification of the truth.

With these conflicts, why persevere? That is what this chapter attempts to address starting with a review of the key features of a successful portfolio management process.

Resource Management

Effective portfolio management should strive to maximize the benefit derived from a limited set of resources. Managers of individual projects managers bemoan what may appear to be a constant lack of resources even in organizations that appear to have few constraints. With unlimited resources, there would be far less incentive for senior management to make hard decisions and little need for portfolio management. Though this might seem to be an ideal state of affairs, it would not drive the efficient use of resources and in real life, there are always limitations. The skills lie in applying those resources that are available creatively and in a way that provides good value. Nevertheless, the resourcing aspects of portfolio management give rise to the commonly held view that it is simply about project prioritization. This is only one aspect of the problem since it also involves achieving balance and aligning projects with the overall business strategy.

Effective resource management is critical if a strategy is to be effectively realized and the problem is not always insufficient resource (i.e., a shortage of skills or capacity). A number of other factors are usually involved, such as

- lack of a clearly defined strategy,
- failure to communicate the strategy to those responsible for delivery,
- lack of imagination with respect to options for efficient application of resources,
- lack of flexibility as to how a project can be resourced (e.g., resistance to use of external suppliers),
- lack of freedom for the project manager to explore and implement creative solutions,
- a cultural style that promotes tension between supply and demand as a means of squeezing more out of the organization, and
- political factors that result in certain projects being favored for reasons that are difficult to justify.

It has been suggested that there are two extremes in the way that projects can be managed. At one end of the spectrum, time is of the essence. The fastest possible plan is presented and resourced as required without detailed interrogation. At the opposite end is the situation where the schedule is constrained by resources that are made available. Too many projects in the first category and the total resource is soon consumed by a relatively small portfolio. Too many in the second may give the appearance of scale but is more likely to result in serial nondelivery. Taking the middle ground for all projects does not usually work either since it can lead to under-achievement in those that may really matter and a tendency to continue to resource less-attractive projects rather than facing up to tough decisions. Though there can be no universally applicable rule, a successful portfolio will often contain a small number (say two or three, depending on the overall scale) "flagship" projects that will be resourced to deliver the fastest possible route to market. For the remainder of the "active" portfolio, there will be a degree of tension, i.e., they could be moved forward more quickly but the strategy is to accept that they will be delayed when resource is limited. The extent of the tension may vary according to the perceived priority of the project but it should always be manageable. There should be very few, if any, projects where resource is so limited that it is difficult to make progress, a scenario that creates a level of frustration for those directly involved and a negative impact in general because it is seen as a wasteful distraction. At its most basic, portfolio management is the process that allows these distinctions to be made in an objective and rational way that can be communicated effectively to stakeholders.

Balance and Strategic Fit

In managing a portfolio, balance is attempted across many dimensions, principally time, risk, return, and resource. One of the many difficulties associated with portfolio management is that these dimensions usually conflict. For example, high-return projects all too often require high resources, involve high risk, and take a long time but, as noted previously, this is where a successful outcome can have a dramatically positive effect on the company as a whole. Failure can also have a negative impact of similar magnitude but, in most established companies, the consequences can be tolerated though the same cannot be said for growth-phase companies. Useful products based on incremental improvements of existing products may still be worthwhile in certain circumstances but only as "fillers" and more likely in emerging companies where they may be seen as a route to early revenues and a way of mitigating risk. What becomes clear is that "balance" is a relative term depending on the status of the company because the factors that will determine whether a particular product "makes sense" will be very different. For an established pharmaceutical company, a product that appears to be of modest value in isolation but allows further exploitation and development of an existing franchise could be justified. For a development-stage company, a product that simply could not be justified in terms of commercial value by a larger organization may be highly significant. Smaller companies seeking an opportunity to demonstrate that they can actually commercialize a product are likely to be looking for niche opportunities that can be marketed cost-effectively. Profit considerations may take second place to the "launch platform" effect; the "we can do this" even if its only a small market. As their is pressure on biotech companies to show that they can create sustainable value increases, there are more outlets for the kind of products that have real medical value but are just not worthwhile in volume terms for the bigger players. So, a project may be of value yet still not be ranked highly if it does not fit with the overall strategic aims of the business, for example, if it does not serve to grow a particular market or sector. Conversely, a project that acts as a stepping-stone to achieving these aims may be given a high priority even if it is not very attractive itself.

Flexibility

Given the above factors, portfolio management would be relatively simple if it were not for uncertainty and change (both internal and external to the business). As a result of this, one of the most important aspects to be included in any portfolio management process is the ability to respond flexibly to a changing environment. In fact, some portfolio strategies would not make sense unless the value of this flexibility is taken into account. Part of the requirement is the anticipation of possible outcomes for a portfolio, the situations these will create, and how to respond to them. Such contingency planning is often talked about but, generally, little time is invested proactively for it. This is in contrast to the amount of time and effort, not all productive, that is expended when an event occurs that perturbs the portfolio. Even though it might have been a predictable event (and many are), the reaction is often one of complete surprise. Frequently, there has been little, if any, preparation for mitigating action and no real consensus on what should be done. The analysis of actions to be taken on one or more follow-up projects should the lead project fail is a good example of how contingency planning can be applied in a portfolio setting. It requires one to think in advance about what might happen, what would be done if it did happen, and what needs to be done in advance to ensure that the contingency plan can be implemented efficiently.

The most important reason for having a portfolio at all is to provide protection in the event of unfavorable business outcomes. This is commonly known as "hedging your bets." This might seem rather obvious but is so important a principle that it is worth repeating. It is one aspect of maintaining flexibility of response. Another aspect is not committing to a course of action prematurely or "keeping all options open." In other words, do not make decisions that commit you to a particular course of action until this is necessary. This is perhaps one of the most important ways of minimizing risk in what is an increasingly uncertain world. On the other hand, this should certainly not be seen as an excuse for inaction, as will be discussed later; a key means of maximizing potential return is to test reasons to kill projects as soon as possible.

The four areas discussed so far represent a considerable challenge but there are further difficulties. One is to design tools and processes that are simple to operate and understand, yet not overly simplistic. Another is to manage the inevitable political, organizational, and logistical problems in operating such a system. These matters are addressed in more detail later in this chapter.

Can Portfolio Management Be Ignored?

Given the problems already outlined, it might be tempting to conclude that portfolio management is simply too complex and too messy to achieve any real benefit. Nevertheless, lack of an effective portfolio management process will lead to

- too many projects chasing too little resources.
- too many mediocre projects starving the few good projects.
- lack of support for business strategy.

On the other hand, an effective portfolio management will support the decision-making process with the minimum of effort in a timely, transparent, and acceptable way. Much more important than this, however, is that it encourages (or even forces) the business at all levels to ask key questions about its portfolio and to formulate appropriate action plans.

PORTFOLIO MANAGEMENT TOOLS

The following section cannot hope to cover all the common tools available for portfolio management in detail but it does give a summary of the major ones and outlines their strengths and weaknesses.

Project Prioritization Methods

As stated previously, portfolio management is not just about prioritizing projects but it is an important aspect nevertheless and the following is a sample of methods which may be used in increasing the order of complexity.

Checklists

For this method, a set of criteria is defined against which all project are evaluated. A project may only proceed if it satisfies all the criteria. This is a very simple and quick technique but is only of real use in quickly culling a range of ideas for future potential projects rather than prioritizing existing ones.

Paired Comparisons

The process here is to compare each project against all the others, one at a time, with the most favorable project scoring 1 and the other scoring 0. Projects may then be ordered, based on total scores. The strength of this technique is that it can easily utilize the "gut feel." Its weaknesses are that the rationale is not explicit and it is very time consuming with a large number of projects.

Dynamic Rank-Ordered Lists

For this process, a set of criteria is defined on the basis of which projects are ranked. For each project, the average criteria ranking is calculated and used to rank it overall. The strengths of this technique are that it is still relatively simple and that the criteria can be chosen to include purely data-driven as well as more-judgmental factors. Its main weakness is that an equal weighting is applied to each criteria; this may not be appropriate.

Weighted Scoring Models

This process overcomes one of the main weaknesses of the dynamic rank-ordered list method since the criteria are each weighted separately. This process is still relatively simple and yet flexible enough to cover a wide range of issues. One of its weaknesses (common to all complex techniques) is that in this process, it is easy to assume a higher level of precision than justified. Another weakness (again in common with most techniques) is that it is difficult to include cross-project relationships. Finally (again common to all techniques), it begs the question "who does the scoring?" If the scoring is done at the project level then a process is required to ensure that it has been done fairly and consistently across all projects. If it is done by a central group then it will require at least some input from projects teams so that they own the final results.

Financial Measures

As with portfolio management techniques, in general, there is no one best financial measure—each simply looks at the project from a different direction. The best way of understanding financial measures is by using a cash flow chart such as that shown in Figure 1. This is a simplified version of real life but it does show the shape of the main costs and sales for a typical pharmaceutical product. In this case, launch is in 2010, peak sales are reached five years later and patent expiry is in 2020. The costs are subtracted from the sales for each year giving the yearly cash flow. This cash flow is then discounted to take into account the fact that money obtained in the future is worth less than today's value. The discounted cash flow is then added up year by year to give the cumulative discounted cash flow. The net present value (NPV) is defined as the cumulative discounted cash flow at a given point in time—in the case of Figure 1 this time point is one year after patent expiry.

The NPV is therefore an attempt to take costs, sales, and the time value of money into account. In general terms, projects with a positive NPV will add value to the business whereas those with a negative NPV will cause the business to lose value and so on a purely stand-alone financial basis should be rejected.

In financial terms, the risk associated with a project may also be measured in several ways. For example, it could be thought of as the money lost up to the next decision point. Alternatively, it could be defined as the money lost should the project fail at launch. An even more conservative approach would be to define it

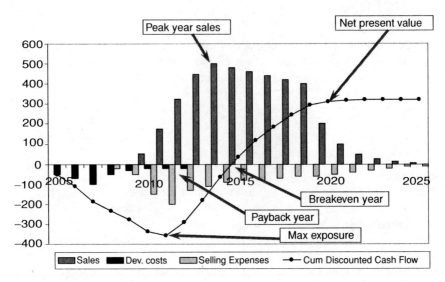

Figure 1   Typical project cash flow chart.

as the maximum amount of money that could be lost. This is sometimes called the maximum exposure or maximum negative discounted cash flow. In Figure 1, this point is reached a few years after launch.

The financial measures mentioned so far have been absolute measures. However, by dividing a return such as an NPV by a cost such as the cost of development, a return-on-investment value may be calculated. This is particularly important when attempting to optimize the use of a resource such as development spending (see later section "Optimizing the Portfolio by Resource and Return").

The strengths of using financial measures are that they are very rigorous and have a strong link to business objectives. One weakness is that it is easy to assume a higher level of precision than justified—financial assessment can encourage an inappropriate attention to detail and can be extremely time consuming. In fact, due to the amount of time and effort taken to provide data for financial analysis, teams often assume that it plays a much more significant part in decision making than is actually the case. Another weakness is that it does not take into account the chance of a project failing at specific points in development. Perhaps the main weakness is that they give only a financial view, which, although important, is nevertheless limited.

Techniques Incorporating Uncertainty

One of the key weaknesses of standard financial assessments is that they take no account of a project failing during development. In practice, however, they can fail at various stages and hopefully before too much money has been spent. This drastically reduces the risks and the average cost of bringing the pharmaceutical products to market and can be taken into account by applying probabilities of

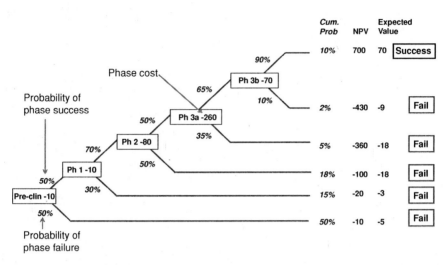

Figure 2 Typical drug development probability tree. *Abbreviation*: NPV, net present value.

success as shown in Figure 2. This allows the calculation of expected NPV that can then be used as a means of prioritizing projects. In this figure, the costs are indicative for a large pharma company, are in million U.S. dollars, and are fully overheaded. They do not, however, include line extension costs. Obviously, these costs may vary widely depending on the type of development and the therapeutic area. The cumulative probabilities for each failed outcome are calculated by multiplying the probabilities of failure of that stage by the probabilities of success of the previous stages. The expected values are then simply the values for an outcome times its cumulative probability. In this example, a US $700 million NPV for the successful outcome has been assumed. In this example, the expected value of success is greater than the expected value of failure and so taking the chances of failure into account is still attractive.

At a further level of sophistication, decision-tree analysis can be used to take into account optional development strategies. For example, such an assessment could include the added value of building in fallback strategies for alternative development should a project fail at a particular stage.

Decision-tree analysis can also be used to explicitly model the effect of one project on another, thus overcoming one of the main shortcomings of all the portfolio techniques mentioned so far. However, at the portfolio level, decision trees rapidly grow in complexity as the number of projects increases. So, although it allows interproject relationships to be analyzed, it is perhaps most useful in exploring options at the project or subportfolio levels.

A technique closely related to decision-tree analysis is option pricing and, in fact, some experts would say both are technically identical. This technique arose in the analysis of financial markets and has proved very popular. Its use in the pharmaceutical industry, however, has been limited due to the complex mathematics generally required.

Optimizing the Portfolio

The key aims of portfolio management are to maximize the value of the launched products with the least use of resources over a sustained period. However, within this broad objective there are many optional strategies. So, "maximizing the value of launched products" may be interpreted as launching a few products with a high average value or a large number of products with a lower average value. Likewise, "with the least use of resources" may mean reducing expenditure on projects through efficiency measures or concentrating on low-risk products, which are less likely to fail in development (or at least fail early). "Over a sustained period" begs the question of how far you can reasonably look and where should the priority lie—short, medium, or long term. The answer that you look as far as you need to sounds very unsatisfactory but to justify research at all implies that it must eventually deliver benefit, which may typically not be for another 15 to 20 years. Of course, this is not to say that you need (or indeed are able) to forecast and plan over that period at a great level of detail but that it must be considered in some form. Again, there will be strategic choices.

Optimizing the Portfolio by Time

Of particular use in analyzing portfolio performance over time are pipeline charts, which show potential launches over time. Such charts are even more insightful when converted to expected values, i.e., the number of launches multiplied by the probability of their occurrence. Such charts, although very simple can have a significant impact on business strategy. Figure 3 compares the expected number of launches based on the current portfolio composition with the current planning assumption and the launches required to meet current business growth objectives. As can be seen, there is a considerable and growing mismatch between these objectives in the medium and long term.

It is worth noting at this point that expected values are much more appropriate at the portfolio level than at the product level. When assessing any individual investment opportunity, a frequent criticism is that the use of probability of launch is not helpful since "it will either launch or it will not." To a certain extent, this is true but the whole point about portfolio management is that when multiple opportunities are available the relative benefits and downsides may be traded off against each other. When looking at the portfolio as a whole, the business needs to know what the average overall performance is likely to be—and this is what expected values tell you.

The expected launches graph may be criticized further in that it only represents one possible view of the future. In practice, we may be luckier (or unluckier) than it suggests. The question then is "what is a reasonable range of possible outcomes?" The answer to this may be explored using a technique known as Monte

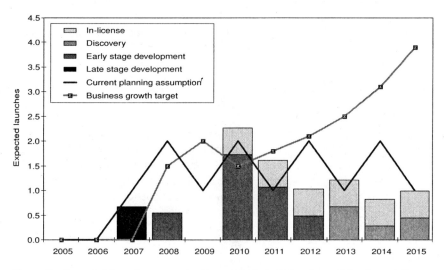

Figure 3 Expected launches versus business growth (split by stage of development).

Carlo analysis. This is a standard statistical technique that allows us to calculate the spread of a range of values.

Figure 4 shows a range of possible future launches. In this case, there is a 50% chance that the number of launches is within the blue band. Beyond the year

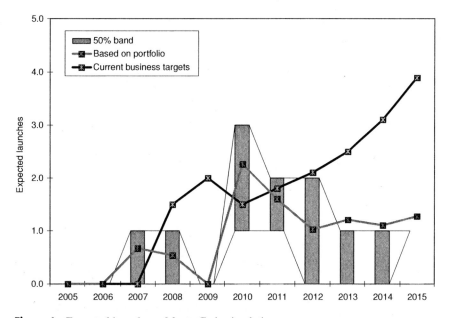

Figure 4 Expected launches—Monte Carlo simulation.

2012, it can be seen that there is a much less than 50% chance that the business would meet the current business strategy in terms of launches. The choice of 50% as the probability defining the width of the band is arbitrary—the calculation could be repeated using any probability but typically is done using 50%, 80%, or 90%. Similarly, graphs of expected sales, profits, and resources are also invaluable.

Optimizing the Portfolio by Risk

Portfolio management would be a relatively trivial problem if the future were certain. Uncertainty is a measure of range of outcomes that may or may not be beneficial. The word "risk" is often used interchangeably (and carelessly) with "uncertainty" but it is helpful to appreciate the distinction between them. Risk can be thought of as the combined likelihood and impact of those outcomes with a negative result. Conversely, outcomes with a positive impact may be thought of as opportunities. There is a danger when carrying out risk assessments and risk management at the project and portfolio level to concentrate mainly on the downsides. However, this may not only undervalue the investment but also be damaging, for example, if product sales are underestimated, this may lead to a situation where production cannot match demand.

Apart from recognizing that uncertainty implies an upside (opportunity) as well as a downside (risk) impact, it is important to remember that risks can, to some degree, be managed. The first step is to recognize and quantify what uncertainties exist. The next step is to develop strategies that

- test key attributes of a product as early as possible.
- generate information that reduces future uncertainty.
- force early failure.
- minimize the damage from negative outcomes (e.g., include fallback strategies).
- maximize the return from positive outcomes (e.g., ensure that capacity exists to take full advantage).

The prime reason for having a portfolio of projects is so that risks can be balanced or "hedged" in financial parlance. A simple way of doing this is to represent projects on a risk matrix as shown in Figure 5.

However, also keep in mind that there are no guarantees!

Optimizing the Portfolio by Resource and Return

Ideally, a business would have, if not unlimited resources, then at least resources that are flexible enough to satisfy whatever varying demands are placed on them. In practice, this is never the case (at least in the short term) and so the portfolio must be balanced to match the resources available. It is also worth noting that in practice, resources can never be used at 100% capacity. This is due to uncertainty in terms of the resources required, either in terms of quantity (the work has been underestimated) or timing (the work takes longer than expected). Another

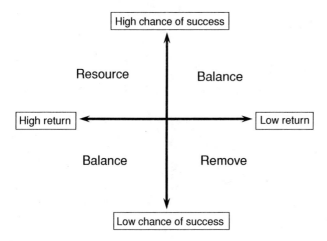

Figure 5   A typical risk matrix.

significant cause of delays, well known to project managers, occurs during decision making at key milestones. It also explains why projects in real life almost invariably take longer than according to the "project template." Modern planning techniques can take this uncertainty into account explicitly but cannot guarantee 100% resource utilization. Instead, these assessments are used to minimize the chances of delay.

    Optimizing the portfolio by resource and return is typically done by ranking projects in terms of some productivity measure (e.g., return divided by investment and then plotting the cumulative return vs. the cumulative investment). This produces a so-called efficient frontier. Figure 6 shows such a plot—cumulative NPV versus cumulative remaining development spending. Two plots are shown—the first represents the existing portfolio and the second represents an enhanced portfolio based on improved development strategies for each of the projects. It can be seen from this graph that for an existing portfolio and level of expenditure (point A), the enhanced portfolio may potentially achieve either the same return for a decreased spending (point B), an increased return for the same spending (point B), or an even higher return for an increased level of spending (point D).

Other Matrix Measures

The previous sections have discussed how the portfolio may be viewed using a limited number of criteria. Figure 7 is an example of how multiple criteria may be combined in one graph. In this case, the vertical axis is a productivity measure [sales over remaining development spending, the horizontal axis is time, and the size of the bubbles is proportional to probability-adjusted value (expected NPV)]. In addition, each bubble has been color-coded—red represents the highest priority

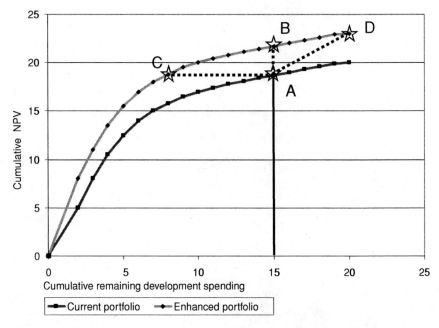

Figure 6 Cumulative return versus cumulative investment. *Abbreviation*: NPV, net present value.

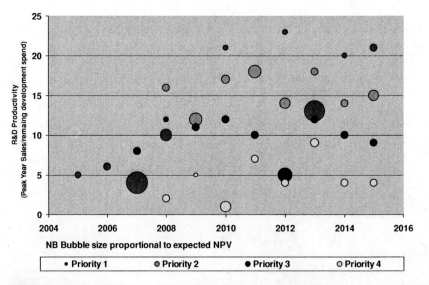

Figure 7 Composite chart.

and yellow the lowest. In this way, the balance of the portfolio can be viewed with respect to time, risk, return, cost, and priority.

There are many other views which may be chosen depending on the particular issues to be addressed, for example:

- fit with corporate strategy,
- durability of competitive advantage,
- cost to project completion,
- time to completion,
- markets/market segments,
- project types (e.g., new, product improvement, product maintenance, cost reduction), and
- technology type.

Conclusion

The choice of tools for portfolio management is dependent on many factors—most of which are related to the company culture rather than any inherent superiority. Indeed, there is no one superior technique and each business must find its ideal compromise in terms of the resource available (time, money, and people), the best balance between judgment and data and between sophistication and practicality. Whatever balance is chosen, the tools used should, at the very least, aid understanding. If possible, they should also add insight. It is truism that a complex model is easier to create than a simple one that addresses key issues and adds insight. However, complex models are difficult to maintain, to explain, and to understand and so may easily be ignored or worse, encourage misleading thoughts. If in doubt, always err on the side of simplicity and remember that even simple tools and tables can help. Figure 8 is an example of a simple portfolio table showing splits by stage of development, customer group, and priority. Such tables have the advantage of being easily understood and so can be used to communicate and discuss the portfolio widely across the organization.

PORTFOLIO MANAGEMENT PROCESSES

Just as with previous sections, the following section cannot hope to cover all the common processes available for portfolio management in detail but it does give a summary of the key issues involved.

Linking Portfolio Management to Strategy

In order for portfolios to meet strategic objectives, all projects within the portfolio and the breakdown of spending across the portfolio must meet these strategic directives. There are two extreme ways of achieving this alignment.

In the top-down approach, resources are allocated to areas of the portfolio and projects are then prioritized within these. A simple example is to define the

	Primary care	Oncology	Specialist
Late development	Proj 1 Proj 2 Proj 11	Proj 14 Proj 15	Proj 26
Early development	Proj 3 Proj 4 Proj 5	Proj 16 Proj 17 Proj 18 Proj 19 Proj 20	Proj 27
Preclinical	Proj 6 Proj 7 Proj 8 Proj 10 Proj 9 Proj 12 Proj 13	Proj 21 Proj 22 Proj 23 Proj 24 Proj 25	Proj 28 Proj 29 Proj 30

Priorities: Red = 1, Green = 2, Blue = 3, Black = 4

Figure 8   Simple portfolio table.

allocation split between early-stage and late-stage development projects and then prioritize these separately.

In the bottom-up approach, projects are considered in detail and prioritized at this level. The strategic fit of projects is addressed by including criteria for strategic fitness into the project-scoring models.

Both of these approaches raise difficulties. The top-down approach begs the question of how resources are allocated and indeed an even more basic question of how strategy is agreed upon. In practice, strategy should be in part influenced by the opportunities available. The bottom-up approach, however, does not address strategy directly but only through a surrogate score which is artificial and opaque.

In practice, a hybrid approach is usually best in which strategy influences project decisions and project opportunities influence strategy. In this way, it is recognized that strategy is not formed in isolation but can and should be influenced by the knowledge of the project teams. Therefore, typically, some general strategic objectives would be set by senior management. Then the individual project teams (often with input from the territorial marketing companies) work to evaluate their projects in an agreed, consistent way. If project teams propose viable options to senior management at this stage then so much the better. These project opportunities are then examined by the senior management and priorities are set. At this stage, the strategic objectives may be modified (e.g., one business area may be allocated higher resources at the expense of another). This process, which is more time and resource consuming than either the purely top-down or bottom-up models, has the great benefits of engaging a much larger section of the organization and recognizing that strategy and portfolio management are dynamic processes. In this way, portfolio management becomes a vital two-way conduit between business strategy formulation and project management.

Portfolio vs. Project Reviews

In a medium to large pharmaceutical company, a typical portfolio process will involve a large number of people over several months which must be carefully planned, managed, and integrated into other business processes. This necessarily means that portfolio reviews must take place at a fixed time of year (typically once or twice a year). Unfortunately, all projects proceed at a different pace, which means that key decision points will rarely coincide with the portfolio review. There is no simple answer to this and sometimes, in extreme cases, some portfolio decisions will have to be delayed until key project information is available.

Portfolios within Portfolios

Simple portfolio management techniques (which are usually the best kind!) often treat each project as being independent. In practice, this is never completely true. For example, projects compete for the same resources (either internally or externally to the company) or may cannibalize one another in the market (which is another way of saying competing for the same customers). A large pharmaceutical company may have several hundred projects in its portfolio, which is too many for anyone to understand in depth all these inter-relationships. For this reason, consideration should be given to smaller groups of projects being considered as a subportfolio at an appropriate level in the company, for example, by therapeutic area or market territory.

Another reason for analyzing subportfolios is to compare like with like. For example, from a risk and financial assessment viewpoint, later-stage projects will usually appear to be far more attractive than those at an earlier stage. It is therefore helpful to consider these two subportfolios separately.

Conclusion

As with the choice of tools, the choice of process for portfolio management is also dependent on many factors. In this case, the choice is even more dependent on company culture rather than any inherent superiority. Again, there is no one superior process and each business must find its ideal compromise in terms of the resource available (time, money, and people), the best balance between judgment and data and between sophistication and practicality.

Whatever process is chosen, it will to a greater or lesser degree be dependent on a large number of contributors at the project level. Each project team will have a vested interest in participating in order to secure resources. Nevertheless, this resource should not be taken for granted. As with tools, it is all too easy to fall into the trap of designing an overly complex process, which, at best, is an irritant and, at worst, a distraction and even demotivates the teams. On the other hand, a

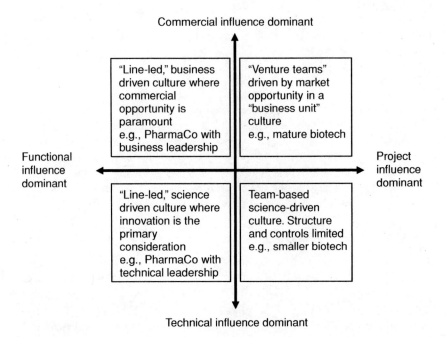

Figure 9 Balance of power for portfolio decisions.

good process is one that supports the decision-making process with the minimum of effort in a timely, transparent, consistent, and acceptable way. Much more important than this, however, is that it encourages (or even forces) the business at all levels to ask key questions about its portfolio and to formulate appropriate strategies.

CUSTOMERS VS. PRACTITIONERS

Portfolio decisions are the responsibility of senior management in most organizations and because of their multifactorial nature, the role is often discharged through a team or committee representative of the various constituencies. These will include heads of functions and heads of project areas, with the balance of power reflecting the underlying culture of the organization (Fig. 9).

For those involved in supporting the portfolio management process, understanding your organization culture and how the process operates are important initial steps toward knowing how to provide valuable input. Whatever the balance, the portfolio management group are the typical consumers of information presented to support portfolio decisions. They have the difficult task of determining the scale and shape of a portfolio that they deem most likely to deliver sustainable value to the business. It is most important that the information provided meets their needs and expectations and is consistent with and supportive of their operating style. No matter how strongly the project teams and portfolio analysts, who are the usual providers of the information, feel that the process could be done more effectively, such a crusading attitude is almost certainly doomed to failure. The reality is that the "customers" in this context will be experienced practitioners with preferred ways of working and there would be the added complication that preferences will not necessarily be uniform for the whole group. The strong recommendation is to spend time understanding what these customers require (or think they require) to improve performance of the portfolio management process. Try to develop approaches and methods that support these perceived needs and even address individual rather than group requirements. For example, certain people will respond better to numerical information whereas others may prefer graphical displays. If some people are contributing less than others, is it because they are not receiving information in a format that they find useful? Ask them and see what can be done.

An overly quantitative approach to portfolio management, exemplified at its extreme by attempts to reduce a complex assessment to a single number, often attracts criticism from those who believe that experience, judgment, and intuition need to be captured in some way. Subjective opinions will always be a factor in decision-making but there needs to be a way of sharing the basis of such opinions so that others can make an input. A dissenting opinion should not automatically be overruled by the majority view—it may be based on knowledge or insight that has not been made generally available and could be a decisive factor. Alternatively, it may be based on erroneous assumptions or prejudices. Either way, the reasons and resultant actions need to be understood. The question is how to capture this "softer" information with sufficient structure to allow valid comparisons and open discussion.

One approach that has been tried with some success is described briefly here. It can complement the more conventional quantitative assessments or be used alone to provide a more qualitative overview. The first step is to agree and describe specific factors that are known to (or could) have an influence on outcome and to group these parameters into sensible clusters. It is then necessary to assess and describe the possible outcomes (up to five) in relation to each factor—from highly negative to highly positive. A "weighting" is applied to each outcome and the general shape of the "curve" agreed (i.e., linear or nonlinear weighting). This information is then transferred to a template and the most useful forms of graphical and/or numerical presentation of the possible outcomes are defined.

This part of the process is best accomplished interactively through a workshop-style session with relevant people under the guidance of one or more facilitators. The time required will vary, depending on the scope and complexity, but might typically range from a half a day (for a relatively contained exercise) to two days. Experience has shown that the quality and the level of ownership of the overall exercise is closely linked to the time and thought given to this customization phase.

PORTFOLIO REVIEW MODEL (EXAMPLE)

	Ref.	*Select the most relevant description by marking with a "x"*				
CLUSTER A:		*Highly Negative*	*Negative*	*Neutral*	*Positive*	*Highly Positive*
PRODUCT ATTRACTIVENESS (Technical)						
Information to support hypothesis	A1	Anecdotal evidence	In vitro experimental data (cell-based or biochemical assays)	In vitro or ex vivo functional data from target organ(s)	In vivo animal data (including xenografts where appropriate)	All previous categories plus supporting human data
Precedent	A2	Speculative - no prior evidence	Sound rationale with limited supporting data	Concept well accepted by peer review	Supportive published data from ongoing development programs	Drugs based on same hypothesis already shown to be effective
Availability of models	A3	None available	Some may be available but details not known	Well-established models available at specialist centres	Well-established models readily accessible on commercial basis	Models available in-house
Status of models	A4	Research concepts	Promising but not yet validated	Validated and generally accepted	Proven, well-controlled and widely published	Industry gold standard
Predictiveness of models	A5	Not known	Equivocal	Generally accepted that results are predictive	Well-documented evidence and supportive peer review	Established track record confirms results are predictive
Nature of models	A6	In vitro only	Ex vivo	In vivo animal model	In vivo animal model with well-defined mechanistic parameters	Human model
Clinical end-points	A7	Likely to require large scale trials to confirm efficacy	Surrogate markers potentially accessible in 'proof of concept' trials but validity of these unconfirmed	Surrogate markers with scientific peer group endorsement available but still to be tested in regulatory setting	Published evidence that proposed surrogate is relevant to target disease state and accessible through small scale trials	Existence of well-characterised, readily accessible surrogate(s) with regulatory endorsement
Regulatory considerations	A8	Regulatory demands not well-defined; likely to be challenging or difficult to satisfy	Regulatory requirements are known but meeting them is likely to be demanding	Regulatory requirement generally understood but not yet tested	Approach can be based on prior examples of success	Well-accepted regulatory requirements with published guidelines and clear pathway
Proof of concept package	A9	Proof of concept would require complex and/or expensive studies	Successful outcome in one or more areas in doubt	Proof of concept possible within context of normal development program	Accelerated proof of concept possible but likely to involve new and unproven concepts that may not be readily accepted	Accelerated package of well-established and accepted manufacturing, analytical, pre-clinical and clinical studies envisaged
		Sub-total				
CLUSTER B:						
MARKET ATTRACTIVENESS						
Volume considerations	B1	Mature market which would be difficult to penetrate	Market not established and growth prospects unclear	Established market with growth potential for new products	Above average market growth predicted (supported by independent forecasts)	Clear demand with independently validated high growth potential
Value considerations	B2	Market dominated by generics with many broadly acceptable products available at low price	New product expected to be relevant to market already available; price premium envisaged	Competitive profile expected to be at least comparable to best in class	Demonstrable evidence of competitive advantage relative to existing product	Few if any products available and demonstrable evidence of competitive advantage
Patent position	B3	Exclusivity through patenting or other means not available and limited opportunity to establish brand strength	Exclusivity through direct patenting or other means not available but novel presentation and strong branding possible	Exclusivity restricted to mode of use only OR one or more major markets likely to be excluded	Robust coverage of compound(s) and applications should be achievable on global basis	One or more granted patents providing good composition of matter coverage in chosen field(s)
Onward licensing/partnership opportunity	B4	No candidates identified	Preliminary discussions held with one or more target licensees	Substantive discussions underway	Term sheet signed	Deal stucture defined and agreement signed
		Sub-total				
CLUSTER C:						
PRODUCT ATTRACTIVENESS (Resource)						
Project in relation to core competencies	C1	Completely new area - sourcing of relevant expertise expected to be difficult	Insufficient in-house capability but sourcing of relevant expertise should be straightforward	Readily managed 'in-house' and contacts known if additional expertise required	Well-qualified to carry out this project based on existing skills and previous experience	Uniquely qualified to carry out this project - no other organisation has the capabilities and contacts
Need for long term support	C2	Significant commitment envisaged to support licensing partner in further development of product	Substantial technology transfer commitment on concluding onward licensing agreement	Specific knowledge-based input for defined period following license deal	Requirement to be 'on call' only for limited period	None envisaged
Downstream considerations (if prospective partner not identified, do not check options marked *)	C3	There is still significant late stage risk associated with product which could compromise successful regulatory approval	Product and/or its proposed use will require significant development effort and/or expertise (e.g. manufacture, clinical trials)	Development and registration requirements expected to be typical for class of product and/or proposed use	*Prospective partner has particular expertise or capacity that will ease later stage development*	*Staightforward development path of which prospective partner has prior relevant experience*
		Sub-total				
CLUSTER D:						
FINANCIAL CONSIDERATIONS						
Estimated peak sales potential	D1	<$100m	$100-250m	$250-500m	$500m-1bn	>$1bn
Estimated development cost to proposed 'exit point'	D2	>$50m	$25-50m	$15-25m	$5-15m	<$5m
Headline deal value envisaged (onward licensing)	D3	<$10m	$10-20m	$20-50m	$50-100m	>$100m
Timing	D4	Royalty only deal >5 years from sales	Royalty and milestone payments yielding <$5m pre-launch	Royalty and milestone payments yielding >$5m but less than $10m pre-launch	Royalty and milestone payments yielding >$10m but less than $25m pre-launch	Royalty and milestone payments yielding >$25m pre-launch
		Sub-total				
		Totals				

The central component of the process takes the form of a structured discussion based closely on the information already developed. "Light-touch" software (the technology element is low-key) is used to capture views, to elicit and consider individual opinions, and to present outcomes. A particular strength of the process is the ability to highlight and discuss the merit of differing and "outlying" opinions rather than simply assuming that the majority or dominant view should prevail. A wide range of factors can be discussed efficiently and the output clustered to provide an easily digestible summary. This is essentially a qualitative process that seeks to capture and assimilate views and opinions and it has the following attributes:

Pragmatism—a simple approach, which captures subjective items very well.
Versatility—can be applied just as easily to "big picture" and detail issues.
Involvement—people-orientated (the whole team can and should contribute).
Ownership—the conclusions are accepted because everyone has had their say.

DECISION MAKING AND CORPORATE CULTURE

What if, after all this, there are still some basic flaws and you think major change is the only answer? The best scenario is when the deficiencies are recognized by a member of the portfolio management group, ideally the leader, and the change process is initiated from within. If this does not happen, some allies will be needed and you will have to canvas opinion. Do not attempt this until you can clearly articulate the deficiencies in an objective way *and* present clear proposals for dealing with them. Bear in mind that if you have been lobbied by project teams, their motivations are likely to be related to getting their project funded. Effective portfolio management, on the other hand, has to be objective and it recognizes that some projects will be given priority over others. Do not fall into the trap of promoting radical change as the only solution— incremental improvements may well deliver what is needed and are likely to more acceptable.

The design and success of any portfolio management process will be determined to a large extent by the preferences of the key decision-making body. Some considerations that should be kept in mind are:

- What are their preferred forms of communication? This can be text, oral, graphical, or tabular and will vary from one member to another.
- What arguments influence them? This will be influenced by the members' function, for example, commercial, technological, financial, mathematical, narrative, scenarios, or models.
- Can they cope with uncertainty? Do they know what they do not know? Do they ask what will the world be or rather what could it be? Are they risk seeking or risk averse? Do they believe uncertainty can be removed with more work, analysis, data, or tools? Are they keen to consider scenarios?

- What are their key drivers? For example, short-term profit versus long-term growth, regional focus versus globalization, and innovation versus marketing?
- How ruthless are they prepared to be? Are they willing and able to kill projects in a timely manner or do decisions tend to be recycled? Is the portfolio full of projects that will not die or even worse, projects that have risen from the dead?
- How far down the organization are they prepared to let key decisions be made? Has the organization devolved decision making to the lowest possible level or are even detailed decisions made at a high level. Related to this is the question of whether they crave detail or are they content with a broad view?
- To what extent do they rely on hard facts versus intuition to support their decisions?

Although a successful portfolio process must be targeted at the key decision makers, it should also open their minds to new ways of thinking since if you cannot change the way they think then you cannot change the way portfolio decisions are made.

KEY MESSAGES

- There is no dominant methodology for portfolio management and the process is often more important than the numbers. There is no mathematical method that can be used to calculate "the right answer." The chosen course of action will be a compromise influenced by a range of factors such as:
  - What are the key issues facing the business?
  - What decisions need to be made?
  - Over what timescale?
  - What are the decision makers' styles?
- These factors will differ from one business to another.
- As in financial evaluation, there is no one right number. Portfolio techniques often concentrate on defining a so-called efficient frontier that shows the optimum composition of a portfolio under various conditions of constraint. For example, one type of frontier may show the portfolios that give the highest return for a given level of risk. Even these methods tend to concentrate on a limited number of project measures and also ignore project interdependencies.
- Portfolio management cannot be ignored but tools and processes must be used with care and with realistic expectations. The simple solution is often the best and will recognize the value of judgment as well as data.
- All portfolios are subject to uncertainty, the source of which may be internal (e.g., project performance) or external (e.g., market conditions). This uncertainty creates risk that must be managed and not ignored. A key strategy for achieving this is to maintain flexibility within the portfolio.
- The design and success of any portfolio management process will be determined to a large extent by the preferences of the key decision-making body and the corporate culture in which they operate.

• A successful portfolio process must be targeted at the key decision makers and should also open their minds to new ways of thinking. If you cannot change the way they think then you cannot change the way portfolio decisions get made.

Perhaps the greatest contribution of portfolio management to the business is that it facilitates or even forces people to talk to each other in a cross-functional and cross-project way and so enhances the organization's portfolio "feel."

SUGGESTED READING

1. Cooper RG, Edgett SJ, Kleinschmidt EJ. Portfolio Management for New Products. Massachusetts, U.S.A.: Persueus Books, Reading, 1998.
2. Dyson RG. Strategic Planning: Models and Analytical Techniques. Chichester, England: John Wiley and Sons, 1992.
3. Steven S. Pharmaceutical Project and Portfolio Management, A report published by Business Insights Ltd., England, 2005.

3

Project Planning: From Basic Concepts to Systems Application[a]

Carl A. Kutzbach
Previously Bayer AG, Wuppertal, Germany

Carole Strong and Sylvia Walker
EXRO Pharma Solutions Ltd., Hertfordshire, U.K.

INTRODUCTION

What Is Planning?

Planning is the process of producing a plan. A good plan optimizes the process to achieve the target objectives of the project in the shortest possible time with the minimum resources. Planning, therefore, means optimizing the classical project management triangle: *performance/time/cost.*

In addition, a plan is an essential means of communication between all project participants to achieve transparency, understanding, and commitment. "Planning makes you free" seems to be a contradiction but, in reality, the efforts devoted to creating a good plan provide the reassurance and freedom of mind that everything that could be reasonably anticipated has been thought of and considered. Of course, unexpected events occur and make it necessary to review and adapt even the best plans.

A plan for developing a drug gives answers to three questions:

- What program of experiments and studies need to be conducted and reported to reach the targeted project performance?

[a] This chapter is based upon the original chapter by Dr. Kutzbach from the first edition and has been revised to reflect contemporary development requirements and planning systems.

- What is the minimum time required to execute this program?
- What resources are required to carry out the work and what is the schedule?

This article will focus on the aspects of performance and time planning. Time optimization planning should assume, initially, that resources are available as and when needed. In the second step, it may be necessary to adapt a plan according to the available resources and existing priorities.

The planning targets of high performance and short development time present a practical conflict. Performance is defined by the quality of the database to ensure rapid and broad registration approval and good positioning in the market. Adding more and larger studies to improve this performance inevitably adds to the time. Late market entry jeopardizes the commercial return because of shorter patent protection and increased risk of an earlier market entry by a competitor with a similar product. A short time to regulatory submission, however, is worthless if approval failure follows or if commercialization is compromised resulting in the need to add studies during the approval process. Planning, therefore, must carefully define the minimum program required to achieve the target without unacceptable risk and also must minimize the time to complete this program.

Differences of Planning in Research and Development

The development of a new therapeutic drug runs through two major phases:

- The research phase of selecting a suitable drug candidate from a large number of compounds screened for activity in vitro or in animal models
- The development phase in which a single compound is carried through the necessary nonclinical and clinical trials required to prove its efficacy and safety and to obtain regulatory approval

During the research phase, the plans for synthesizing new compounds are constantly adapted to the outcome of the screening assays. Long-term planning in this phase is therefore largely restricted to the overall scope of time and resources applied to the project. This work is managed by the disciplines of chemistry and experimental biology within the research and discovery function.

In the development phase, however, the contributions of many disciplines must be closely coordinated to minimize the time to interim decision points and to the final project completion.

This article will focus on the planning of development projects. Planning is facilitated by the fact that regulatory guidelines and directives are often available to help in designing the development program for a particular disease indication. Generally, development is structured in the phases shown in Table 1.

Planning of the development process is essentially a stepwise, continuous process starting with a defined target and ending with a detailed plan of action. The plan will be continuously adapted in the light of development findings and changing circumstances as shown in Table 2.

Table 1 Standard Phases of Drug Development

Phase	Start	Main tasks	End	Average duration (mo)
Preclinical	Development decision	Safety evaluation in animals; laboratory and initial scale-up of API; drug product formulation for phase 1	Approval to treat first human subject	15
1	Start of first tolerability and kinetic study in humans	Safety, tolerability and kinetics in humans; extended toxicology; API process development; drug product optimization/ manufacture for phase 2; establishment of clinical database	Approval to start first therapeutic trial	12
2	Start of first therapeutic trial	First proof of therapeutic efficacy; determination of effective dose; long-term toxicology	Approval to start large pivotal therapeutic trials	24
3	Start of first large pivotal trial	Statistical proof of efficacy and safety in a large, diverse patient population; API and drug product scale-up and validation; compilation of regulatory dossier	Completion of documentation for electronic regulatory submission	30
Approval	Submission in first country	Response to questions and requests of regulatory authorities; production of launch supplies; premarketing and sales force training	Marketing approval	12–48

Abbreviation: API, active pharmaceuticals ingredient.

THE BASIS OF THE PROJECT PLAN

Defining the Project Target

Each plan describes the route to a target. A good plan requires and helps to clarify an exact definition of the target. The general target of drug development is an

Table 2   Steps in the Planning Process

1. Define the target
2. Prepare a list of necessary work packages (studies)
3. Determine the logical sequence and estimate durations
4. Determine the critical path
5. Optimize the plan to reduce critical path length
6. Plan resources and costs and adjust for resource and budget constraints and priorities
7. Adjust plan during execution to new data, as required

approved and commercially successful drug product. Drug performance targets are commonly described by the target indication and the route of administration. This is further specified in terms of efficacy, safety, and patient convenience parameters. Parameters such as socioeconomic benefit, unique selling proposition, and maximum cost of goods may be added. Early in the development process, some companies use draft (patient information) PI-sheets covering most of these parameters. Others start with a less detailed target product profile (sometimes also called project target profile or similar). In any case, it is essential that the efficacy and safety parameters are defined as quantitatively as possible so that they can serve as design parameters for clinical studies. Of course, the minimum requirements must describe a product that has a good chance to be competitive when entering the market several years in the future. If these minimum requirements are not met in the study program, then discontinuation of the project must be considered (see example of a target product profile in Fig. 1).

Often a development candidate offers the opportunity for development in more than one therapeutic indication or in different formulations. These constitute different subprojects that require their own fully detailed target profiles.

Prior to the initiation of the planning process, the selection of subproject(s) to be developed initially and those that present options for future line extensions or licensing opportunities should be made. A parallel development of all possible options, in most cases, would require too many resources and increase considerably the development time to first marketing approval. The selection of the target for the first development may be based on the chance for clinical success, on an expected shorter time to market, or on other valid reasons. Parallel development of two indications is made easier if they use the same formulation and therefore can use the same nonclinical and phase 1 program. On the other hand, the potential of consecutive or combination therapy by intravenous and oral routes may be important enough to justify its parallel development, for example, with certain antibiotics.

If broad international registration and marketing are intended, it must also be investigated if identical targets are appropriate in all countries or regions. There are significant differences in medical practice, definition of indications, and acceptance of application routes by the patient in different regions to be taken into account. The intent must be to cover as much as possible with a shared core program and studies added for specific local requirements wherever necessary.

Project Target Profile				
Project: **AZ 1000** Indication: **Hypertension**		Date: Formulation: **Tablet**		
Project Attributes		**Realization**		
All attributes are minimum requirements	Quan- titative	cer- tain	pro- bable	not clear
1. Efficacy				
* Significant responder rate (long-term treatment)	>60%		*	
* Dose dependant efficacy			*	
* One well-tolerated dose should reduce diastolic blood pressure at trough compared to placebo by	>8 mm Hg		*	
2. Tolerability				
* Risk/benefit ratio and incidence of adverse events at least comparable to ACEIs or Ca antagonists e.g.:				*
metabolically neutral			*	
no narrow therapeutic index			*	
no negative effects on electolyte balance				*
no restrictions when combined with common drugs,			*	
particularly CV and MD			*	
no major contraindications				
no CNS side effects				
* (a) in contrast to Ca antagonists no clinically relevant peripheral edema or increase in heart rate				
* (b) in contrast to ACE inhibitors no negative impact on lung (particularly no cough induction) and those renal conditions negatively affected by ACE inhibitors				
3. Convenience			*	
* Once-a-day application		*		
* Small, easy to swallow oral formulation				
4. Innovation (USP)				*
* Demonstration of 2a) or 2b) without additional adverse effect				

Figure 1   Example of a possible format for a project target profile.

Legal and Regulatory Requirements

The plan must also take into account government laws, guidelines, and points to consider of the regulatory authorities in the target countries as well as rules of ethical committees or institutional review boards (IRBs). If clear guidelines do not exist, it is useful to obtain the advice of key opinion leaders in the field, for example, on choosing therapeutic targets and clinical end points. Furthermore, every opportunity to present the plan to a regulatory authority should be taken to obtain its opinion or consent.

PREPARING THE PROJECT PLAN

Elements of a Project Plan

The basic building block of any project plan is the single task leading to a defined result, commonly known as a work package. The defined result is usually a study report required for regulatory clinical trial application (CTA), investigational new drug (IND), new drug application (NDA), marketing authorisation application (MAA) submission. It may, however, also be a development or marketing plan or a produced and released batch of drug substance or formulation. For many work packages in drug development, the scope of study and content of the report are clearly defined by regulatory guidelines or by internal company standards. A list of all work packages and their definitions is an essential prerequisite for a standard plan. In addition, the department involved in carrying out the work should be specified. If several departments contribute to a single work package, the responsible department should be identified. There should also be a standard time estimate for executing the work package in the absence of resource constraints and abnormal technical problems.

Often, it is useful to break larger work packages down into smaller tasks, commonly called jobs. Again, each such job must have a defined end point. A simple example is a sequence such as a protocol design, treatment period, and data evaluation and reporting in clinical or toxicological studies. Other job structures may be more complex, such as the many individual experimental studies comprising the technical or analytical IND or NDA documentation packages for a drug substance or a drug product. A list of jobs for each work package serves as a checklist and facilitates definition.

There is considerable flexibility in defining larger or smaller work packages and jobs within these definitions. Two general rules may be useful for practical planning:

1. Work packages should, preferably, be carried out within a single function.
2. Work packages identify the level of planning and time tracking by the project manager whereas jobs are tracked within the functions responsible for the work package.

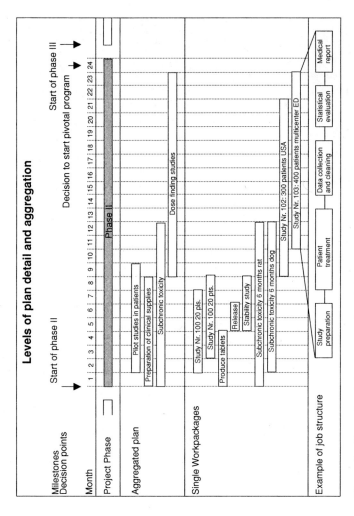

Figure 2 Example of plan presentations in increasing levels of detail.

Using these definitions, the size of work packages may vary in different companies depending on the agreed distribution of project-tracking responsibility between project management and line functions. Nevertheless, some common practices have evolved and a typical project plan contains about 200 to 300 work packages.

For senior management presentation and review, a plan containing all work packages is much too detailed and needs focusing by aggregation. The first level of aggregation may be the combination of individual studies in one discipline into a super work package for each phase such as all toxicological or animal pharmacokinetic studies in preclinical phase, the basic clinical phase 1 program, or all clinical studies in phases 2 and 3. The most condensed plan for practical use is obtained by aggregating all activities into the standard development phases. An example of the different detail levels of planning is given in Figure 2.

The project plan should also be structured by using defined decision points and milestones. Decision points indicate the requirement for a management decision to enable continuation of the project. The decision is typically based on an evaluation of completed studies, a commercial evaluation of the project, and a plan covering at least the next project phase. The scope and level of detail of these decision prerequisites must be carefully defined. Milestones are easily measurable time points of project progress. They serve for planning and comparison of progress to plan. A set of practical milestones and decision points is given in Table 3.

The First Plan

Generally, conceptual planning should be done from the end to the beginning, starting with the outline of the pivotal clinical trials necessary for approval and then adding the nonclinical, clinical dose-finding, and clinical pharmacology studies

Table 3 Proposal of Milestones and Decision Points

Milestones	Project phase	Decision
1. Project presentation 2. Application for IND/CTA	Preclinical	1. Start development 2. Start clinical trials
3. Start phase 1	Phase 1	
4. Start phase 2	Phase 2	
		3. Start pivotal program
5. Start phase 3	Phase 3	
6. Clinical cutoff		4. Submit for approval
7: Submission of NDA/MAA 8: Approval of NDA/MAA	Approval	5. Launch
	Prelaunch	
9: Launch		

Abbreviations: IND, investigational new drug; CTA, clinical trial application; NDA, new drug application; MAA, marketing authorisation application.

Table 4 Tasks in Preclinical Development

Safety evaluation	
Toxicology	Repeat oral- or IV-dose studies in one rodent and one nonrodent species duration from 2 wks up to 3 mo Mutagenicity tests Reproduction toxicology
Safety pharmacology	Effects on cardiovascular, respiratory, gastrointestinal, renal, and CNS systems
Pharmacokinetics/metabolism	Basic kinetics and single dose ADME in 2 species; autoradiographic distribution pattern; protein binding Metabolism in vitro; toxicokinetics
Production	
API preparation and scale-up	Scale-up from laboratory to pilot scale to produce necessary amounts for phase 1 under GMP conditions; last chemical conversion step should preferably be finalized
Drug product development	Formulation with suitable stability and acceptable bioavailability for phase 1 studies

Abbreviations: ADME, absorption, distribution, metabolism, excretion; GMP, good manufacturing practice.

that are prerequisites to enter the large and final studies. The initial preclinical development phase, however, typically follows a fairly standardized path and therefore may be planned and started before a complete project plan has been finalized. The main tasks of the preclinical program are shown in Table 4. The early development will be designed after a careful review of the preclinical research data. Furthermore, the intended therapeutic use is taken into account for finalizing the toxicological study plan with regard to the choice of species and treatment duration.

The first outline of the project plan will usually be a list of nonclinical and clinical studies with their estimated durations and logical dependencies (Table 5). A simple graphical representation of these data will show which sequence of activities determines the critical path of the project and its minimum total duration (Fig. 3). Then, milestones and decision points are added on the time axis. A standard plan is a very useful tool for the project manager to check for the completeness of this first plan and to obtain initial time estimates. However, these must be confirmed later or adjusted depending on resource availability and agreement with the group carrying out the task.

It is advantageous to complement the list and time schedule with a narrative describing the assumptions and rationale underlying the plan. In particular, this should refer to the guidelines and regulations considered. The narrative should also point out which plan details are considered preliminary and need further information for finalizing. It may also be useful to document the reasons for major deviations from the standard plan.

Table 5 Essential Elements of a First Plan

Study description	Comment	Result required for item	Estimated duration (wks)
1. Clinical studies			
1.1. Basic phase 1 studies	Basic tolerability and kinetics in increasing single and multiple doses. May include pharmacodynamic monitoring	1.3	30
1.2. Extended phase 1 studies	Interaction, bioequivalence, human mass balance, QTc study in volunteers, special patient groups	1.5, 8.2	52
1.3. Proof-of-concept efficacy trial	This may include pharmacodynamic monitoring in 1.1	1.4	32
1.4. Dose-finding clinical trials (phase 2)			
	Example: 2 studies with 300 patients, 2 mo treatment	1.5	72
1.5. Pivotal phase 3 efficacy trials	Example: 2 studies with 500 patients, 3 mo treatment	8.2	120
1.6. Long-term safety trials			
	Number of patients and duration according to guidelines and therapeutic area	8.2	120
1.7. Special studies	Depending on therapy class and marketing requirements, e.g., special populations	8.2	26–104
2. Toxicological studies			
2.1. Acute toxicity		1.1	8
2.2. Repeat-dose toxicology	2 or 4 wks in 2 species including dose-range finding	1.1	24
2.3. Additional repeat- dose toxicology	3 mo in 2 species	8.2	26
2.4. Long-term repeat dose toxicology	6 mo in rodent and 9 mo in nonrodent species	8.2	70
2.5. Reproduction studies	Embryotoxicity—2 species, includes dose-range finding	1.2, 1.3	36
	Fertility, peri/postnatal toxicity	1.4	22

Table 5 (*cont.*)

Study description	Comment	Result required for item	Estimated duration (wks)
2.6. Carcinogenicity	Lifetime studies in mice and rats	8.2	150
2.7. Mutagenicity	Selection from several in vitro and in vivo tests	1.1–1.4	14
3. ADME/pharmacokinetic studies			
3.1. Pre–phase 1 package	Example: basic kinetics (2 species), single-dose ADME (2 species); autoradiographic distribution, metabolism in vitro; protein binding	1.1–1.4	26
3.2. Extended studies	Example: repeated dose ADME, placental transfer, metabolism in vivo, excretion into milk, enterohepatic circulation in rat and one nonrodent	1.5–8.2 (earlier in Japan)	52
4. Safety pharmacology			
4.1. Basic package evaluating vital systems	Example: hERG channel, Purkinje fiber, cardiovascular and respiratory evaluation in vivo, neurobehavioral Irwin screen	1.1	18
4.2. Extended studies			
(Requirement/timing is dependent on therapeutic area)	Example: renal function, GI function, drug dependence/abuse potential	1.4–8.2	26
4.3. Additional studies	Example: safety pharmacology of metabolites	8.2	26–52
5. API manufacturing			
5.1. Laboratory API synthesis and analysis		6.1	12
5.2. GMP synthesis and analysis		6.1	14
5.3. GMP process optimization and development	Long-term repeat dose toxicology should use API by final route of manufacture	2.4, 6.3	26

(cont.)

Table 5   *(cont.)*

Study description	Comment	Result required for item	Estimated duration (wks)
5.4. Final process validation	Validated production scale process	6.5, 8.2	52
6. Drug product manufacturing process			
6.1. Preclinical formulation		2.1–2.6	2–14
6.2. Phase 1 GMP formulation	A simple formulation, e.g., nonblended API in a loose-filled capsule or a drinking solution	1.1	12
6.3. Drug product optimization/manufacture phase 2	Ideally should be final formulation	1.4	22
6.4. Phase 3 manufacture		1.5	26–104
6.5. Drug product scale-up and validation		8.2	26–104
7. Analytical			
7.1. API physicochemical evaluation	Including method development	8.1, 8.2	10–52
7.2. Formulation characterization	Including method development	8.1, 8.2	10–52
7.3. Stability of API		8.1, 8.2	≥ 52
7.4. Stability of clinical formulation	Sufficient to support length of clinical program	8.1, 8.2	≥ 52
7.5. Stability of final formulation	Sufficient to support intended shelf life	8.1, 8.2	≥ 104
8. Regulatory			
8.1. Clinical trials submission (CTA/IND)		1.1	4
8.2. Marketing approval submission (MAA/NDA)	Accelerated approvals may be considered in less time, e.g., 26 wks		52

Abbreviations: QTc; ADME; hERG, human ether-a-go-go; API, active pharmaceutical ingredient; GMP; CTA; IND.

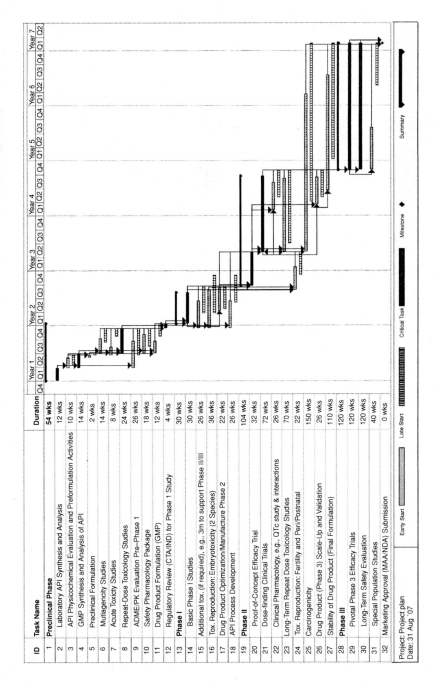

Figure 3 First project plan drawn as Gantt chart showing critical path and buffer times for noncritical activities (prepared using Microsoft Project®). *Abbreviations*: API, active pharmaceutical ingredient; GMP; ADME; PK, pharmacokinetics; CTA; IND; QTc; MAA; NDA.

Optimizing the Plan

The first plan may result in an unacceptably long total development time. Optimization strategies including the possibility of parallel work and task overlap should now be explored. In other parts, it may also be too optimistic because some prerequisites were overlooked or do not agree with current regulations.

Consequently, plan optimization, above all, should address the completeness of the plan and shortening of the critical path; this can be facilitated by an experienced project manager. The project manager must ask the right questions and insist on a thorough evaluation aimed at shortening the critical path. Although safety and ethical reasons prescribe a consecutive and stepwise performance of preclinical and clinical studies, considerable flexibility for refinement exists. Much of the potential for time reduction is in the evaluation phase of studies. However, it is often not necessary to evaluate all data before taking the decision to start the next study. The following are examples of typical questions to be addressed in plan optimization:

a. Completeness of plan
   - Have all relevant guidelines been identified and their content been considered?
   - Do the studies address all product performance statements within the target product profile?
   - Have all local requirements for the target countries been investigated and considered?
   - Have marketing requirements been defined and incorporated?
   - Have all necessary data and qualitative and quantitative material prerequisites for each study been planned with sufficient lead time?
b. Shortening of the critical path
   - Are all work packages on the critical path essential for the start of their successors or can some be completed independently?
   - What is the minimum output of each critical path study before its successor can be started? Examples:
     ○ What is the duration of toxicological exposure required prior to the start of phase 1?
     ○ Which phase 1 studies should be completed before starting the phase 2 program, i.e., drug interaction study?
     ○ Can initiation of phase 3 be based on interim analysis of phase 2 studies rather than their final evaluation?
     ○ What stability-supported shelf life of the formulation is needed before the start of a particular study?
     ○ Where are final quality-checked reports necessary for continuing the project and where is a draft report sufficient?
     ○ How can the study evaluation be expedited, for example, by concurrent or remote data entry?

○ Is it possible to increase the assumed patient enrollment rate to reduce the clinical phase of a study?

○ Which task is likely to overrun the estimated duration because of unexpected technical problems and can this risk be reduced by adding resources early?

In the optimization phase, standard duration estimates for work packages are replaced by realistic calendar start and finish dates. The activities to be carried out by respective functions can be scheduled with reasonable reliability for the following one- to two-year time frame. If resources in the required time window are limited, the possibilities of adding resources or external contracting should be considered early.

Published benchmarks of development phase durations can serve as a measure to indicate whether the time lines of a plan are aggressive or comfortable. Real development times show wide variations. Some of this is caused by different study requirements for different indications or by particular experimental or technical problems with the development compound. However, some companies show consistently shorter development times than others, which is probably indicative of good project planning and management. Table 6 lists some benchmark data from various sources. An aggressive development plan must aim for a duration at the lower end of this list because the durations shown in Table 6, in many cases, reflect delays resulting from unexpected problems that always occur in practice.

Additional timesaving possibilities may be achieved by conducting feasibility studies ahead of the selection of territories for phase 2/3 clinical programs.

Another interesting option is to use the cold season in the Southern Hemisphere for an anti-infective study instead of waiting for the next winter in the North.

The following sections are further practical examples of the necessary considerations and decisions for different tasks within the development process.

Table 6 Reported Clinical Development Phase Durations for Compounds in Development for Chronic Indications During 1990–1992 in Months

	Europe			Japan			U.S.A.		
	Range	Mean	n	Range	Mean	n	Range	Mean	n
Phase 1	6–26	15	14	6–13	12	5	6–20	11.5	8
Phase 2	12–40	27	13	21–37	28	5	12–60	24	8
Phase 3	21–76	38	10	24–73	32	5	28–48	34	9

Source: Centre for Medicines Research (CMR) report CMR94–6R, The Strategy and Management of Successful Global R&D, August 1994; CMR poster presented at the Drug Information Association 30th Annual Meeting, June 5–9, 1994, Washington, D.C.

Toxicology and Safety Investigations

Existing guidelines allow considerable flexibility in designing the toxicological program with regard to species selection, duration, and sequence of studies. The ideal species are those in which pharmacokinetics and metabolism are most similar to humans. Unfortunately, human data are not known at the beginning and an intelligent choice may only be made based on some structural similarity to drugs investigated earlier. Therefore, most initial studies are done with the standard species—rat and dog. However, human kinetic and metabolism data should be collected as early as feasible to make the most appropriate choices of species for long-term studies. The required duration of toxicological studies is determined by the intended treatment duration. For short treatment courses up to four weeks, as with most antibiotics, three-month toxicological studies are sufficient for the clinical program and approval.

It is good common practice to determine target organs and appropriate dose levels in short-term or smaller pilot studies before embarking on the more costly long-term studies. However, the risk of missing the appropriate dose range can also be minimized by using more than the required minimum three doses in a study. A further option is to add additional animals to a long-term (e.g., six-month) study and perform an interim kill to get an early indication that the study is on the right track. However, for ethical reasons, the toxicological program should be designed to avoid unnecessary repetition of studies with large numbers of animals. Generally, the most efficient toxicological program for a particular drug development should be planned by the toxicological expert with input by the whole project team rather than following a traditional standard pattern.

There is evidence that over the decade from 1992 to 2002, drug development times were progressively reduced (1). This is seen clearly when the clinical trial phase (IND to NDA) and regulatory review period are reviewed year after year based on the IND opening year. While over the whole period the median time for clinical trials and the regulatory review phase was 5.1 years and 1.2 years respectively for the 168 drugs in the database, the median times for more recently developed drugs was shorter such that for INDs opening in 1993 to 1995, the median total time for both clinical and regulatory phases was under 5 years. However, as discussed in chapter 6, there is also evidence that this trend has not persisted and may indeed be reversed.

Phase 1 Studies

The main objective of phase 1 studies is to establish the safety and tolerability of a new drug in healthy human volunteers. Initially, a single dose, one to two orders of magnitude below the no-effect dose in animals, will be administered with incremental dose increases and careful measurement and observation of a large number of laboratory and clinical parameters. Several such steps may be required until therapeutic drug levels are reached. After establishing single-dose tolerability, this will be repeated in multiple-dose studies whose treatment duration depends on the intended therapeutic dosing scheme. The total duration of this program depends greatly on the time required to evaluate a completed study sufficiently to justify initiating the next step. This can be done most efficiently if the whole sequence of studies is undertaken in the same institution and by the same investigator. In addition to safety information, many other valuable data are derived from phase 1 studies. Pharmacokinetic measurements give critical information on bioavailability and half-life that are often very different from the animal data. This is an important early guidance for formulation development. A low oral bioavailability of a costly drug substance may jeopardize the commercial success of a project unless a formulation with improved bioavailability can be developed. Low bioavailability also carries an increased risk of safety problems because of larger interindividual variations. If marketing considerations require a once-daily dosing and a short half-life makes this unlikely, the development of controlled release formulations should be started early. Companies are now increasingly designing their phase 1 programs to collect pharmacodynamic information, relevant to the intended therapeutic use, from healthy subjects, whenever possible. For example, bronchoprovocation or challenge studies give an important indication of the efficacy of asthma drugs. It may even be possible to determine the effective dose range with sufficient accuracy so that pivotal efficacy studies may be started immediately, parallel to formal dose-finding studies, with considerable saving in total development time. Careful judgment by clinical experts is required in such decisions.

Several nontraditional approaches, including microdosing, are being explored to obtain early assessment of pharmacokinetic and pharmacodynamics in first–in-human studies. These methods may help early drug development decisions to be made more efficiently (2).

Clinical Development

Clinical development is the subject of a specific chapter in this book. Therefore, only a few general comments will be given here. The duration of clinical studies determines most of the critical path for the largest part of the development program and initially planned times for completing studies are often exceeded because estimated enrollment rates were too optimistic and countermeasures to prevent further delays were started too late. Important choices to be made, especially by companies doing parallel international development, are the country or continent for the study and whether to perform it through its own organization or contract it totally or in part to a clinical research organization. In an international development effort, common understandings of goals and good coordination of activities between the regional departments are prerequisites for efficiency. Study sizes must be carefully calculated to offer the necessary statistical power for detecting the minimum therapeutic effect compatible with the approval criteria for a commercially viable product. In drug comparison studies, special attention must be given to the choice of the most suitable comparative drug. Different comparative drugs may be required in different regions or countries. Some of the most spectacular progress in reducing total drug development time has been made by shortening the time for trial data evaluation through continuous and/or remote entry of data during the study. In particular, this applies to interim analyses that may allow the next consecutive study to start earlier, when, for example, the effective dose range is sufficiently well established. The price for this faster study evaluation, however, is more work in the study planning and setup phase, which therefore must be started early enough. The full benefit of a rapid study evaluation is obtained only when the next study is ready to start immediately. For this purpose, the design and preparations must also be as flexible as possible to allow for some last-minute adjustments. For example, additional dose strengths of the formulation may be manufactured and stocked to avoid delays by a late change in the dosing scheme.

Manufacturing Development

Generally, clinical and toxicological studies are the most time consuming and, typically, are the critical path activities of drug development. They also carry the highest risk of negative outcomes leading to project delay or even termination. However, drug substance and drug manufacturing issues are becoming increasingly complex and need careful attention in planning. Reasons for this include

- progression of more complex chemical structures—often stereoisomers— leading to larger number of synthesis steps and increased manufacturing costs.
- increased demand for controlled release or other special formulations.
- more stringent regulatory requirements for GMP manufacturing, for example, following the Clinical Trials Directive, 2004, GMP manufacturing is required for all phase 1 clinical formulations.
- biological agents, usually proteins, have extended lead in times for synthesis.

Newly developed technologies for advanced formulations often require lengthy optimization and scale-up, with considerable risk of unexpected problems and resulting delays. Every effort has to be made to use the final formulation in the large-scale, pivotal, phase 3 trials. Final formulation means that this formulation is supported by a sufficiently validated manufacturing-scale process and sufficient stability data to minimize the need for further optimizations leading to the risk of changed properties. This rule is especially important for controlled release formulations because almost every formulation change requires a proof of bioequivalence with its inherent high risk of failure and the consequent repetition of clinical trials. For example, if development of the final formulation determines the initiation of phase 3 clinical development, the risk of repetition of study must be carefully assessed against the later availability of decision-relevant data caused by waiting for the final formulation.

A positive development in recent years has been a trend to shorter regulatory approval times, both in the United States and in Europe. With current NDA/MAA approval times coming out to be sometimes less than one year, companies must be ready for preapproval inspections within three months after submission. To avoid launch delays after approval, production scale-up of active pharmaceutical ingredient (API) and drug product (including validation batches) and commercial manufacturing preparation activities to supply the forecasted market penetration must be conducted parallel to phase 3 trials.

Another reason for the early selection of the final formulation is the need to complete stability studies in time to support the approval and the intended shelf life at launch. Achievement of these tasks may also require earlier investments at a time when the efficacy and long-term safety of the new drug are still under evaluation. The investment risk can be minimized if the company owns a multi-purpose manufacturing plant capable of supplying the market for the first two to three years after launch.

Several previous examples have demonstrated that starting new activities before the results of preceding studies are fully evaluated carries the increased risk that studies might be repeated because of inappropriate design. This risk must be carefully assessed against the opportunity of increased development speed. Alternative scenarios of outcomes and their consequences should be carefully considered and modeled during the planning process. In many cases, it is advantageous to focus the plan on a go/no-go decision and to reach this in the shortest possible time with the minimum amount of effort and data. If the outcome is negative, this allows the most efficient use of resources. In the event of a positive signal, the missing studies can be started quickly without much loss in total time. The exact strategy selected will be specific to the project.

Stepwise Planning and Decision Points

In view of the acknowledged uncertainties in drug development, effort would be wasted to plan the project from beginning to end in full detail. Over a 10-year period ending in 2000, only approximately 11% of compounds tested in humans across 10 large pharmaceutical companies were eventually approved for marketing in the United States and/or Europe (3). It is sufficient to plan the work for the next phase or to the next major decision point in full detail by defining each work package, its duration, prerequisites, resource requirements, and the departments/persons responsible for its execution. For the subsequent phases, an estimate of total time required should be made based on a listing of major, necessary studies, their sequence, and standard durations. The current trend to invest in biotechnology companies raises the profile of detailed plan and cost projections to specified milestones, this being required for presentation to both the investment community and potential licensing partners.

Additional project-specific decision points should be defined for recognized or probable critical issues so as not to waste resources on projects with a limited chance of success. The project plan should aim to obtain the data for such decisions as early as possible even if the overall critical path analysis allows for later investigations. Examples:

- Potential for toxicity highlighted from structural alerts within the molecule (e.g., phototoxicity or mutagenicity)

- Feasibility of achieving the defined, unique selling propositions
- Feasibility of a commercially acceptable cost of goods
- Feasibility of achieving bioavailability for an oral formulation
- Feasibility of once-daily dosing, if required for marketing reasons
- Feasibility of achieving an adequate shelf life

Some of these or other decision points may lead to a clear go/no-go decision. Minimum performance requirements must be defined in advance; depending on possible outcomes, several alternative courses of action may be possible. Scenario-type plans must be prepared to determine the impact on total project time, commercial value, and resource requirements.

The Management of the Planning Process

Pharmaceutical development involves many disciplines and functions. Planning, therefore, is best done as a team effort with representatives from all the functions, led by an experienced, independent project manager. The functional representative's task is to define the methods, protocols, and study outlines required for the necessary proofs of efficacy, safety, and technical feasibility. Responsibility for making schedule commitments for the work packages and ensuring availability of needed resources should be addressed. The project manager's role is to focus on the project target, overall time lines, and efficient use of resources ensuring that nothing is overlooked and that the contributions of the different disciplines is coordinated with the minimum amount of delay and with as much parallel work as feasible. One of the project manager's prime responsibilities is to ensure that every person involved in the project has the information necessary for contributing in the best and most timely manner. This becomes essential when working within the virtual project team environment.

The whole team should discuss every aspect of the plan in detail to address all potential impacts of a particular experimental design or the "knock-on" effect of slippage of activity time lines in one area on the tasks under the responsibility of another department. The regulatory consequences of changes, such as those in study protocols or in formulation composition, must be carefully addressed to prevent later delays resulting from the need to repeat or include additional studies. These considerations also apply to plan adjustments in response to technical or organizational problems that the executing department too often considers solely its own responsibility.

Alternative scenario planning encourages frank and creative discussions amongst team members allowing cross-fertilization of ideas between disciplines. Ready access to the plan electronically enables transparency to all stakeholders and promotes ownership. It is essential to have strict version control of shared plans to maintain effective communication.

For duration and completion planning of work packages, the project manager must, in principle, rely on the estimates given by the responsible team member. The project manager, however, should investigate the potential for time reduction, especially if the activity is on the critical path and if the estimate is significantly longer than the duration given in the standard plan. In an optimized plan, it is normal that many work packages are very close to the critical path, i.e., their buffer times are only a few weeks or even days. Delayed start or small delays in their execution may quickly put them on the critical path. Therefore, it is essential that the project team and the project manager give the same attention to these activities as to the true critical path activities. Whenever possible, these activities should begin on the early start date, and any indications of a threatening delay must be quickly communicated and acted upon.

PLANNING TOOLS AND SYSTEM SUPPORT

Network Plans

The concept of network plans was developed in parallel with general project management systems and is often wrongly taken as the essence of project management. Network plans are an extremely useful tool to organize most project activities so that the influence of time changes in each activity and the overall project completion time is clearly visible. The key output of a network plan is the critical path, the sequence of activities that determines the minimum duration of the project. It also defines lag times or buffers for all other activities. Reduction of the time to completion is possible only by doing critical path activities quicker or by rearranging the work so as to do activities in parallel instead of in sequence. Tracking of time must focus primarily on critical path activities (Fig. 4).

The Standard Plan

Pharmaceutical development of different drug candidates follows a broadly similar course, largely set by scientific method and regulatory requirements; a formal "standard or generic plan" is a very helpful tool. It summarizes the knowledge, experience, rules, and definitions of a development organization and serves as a template and checklist for new project plans. Its main value is to provide a repository for a project plan capturing pivotal activities and enabling customization for each individual project based upon the considerations outlined in the previous sections.

Standard plans are normally in the form of an integrated network plan, showing all activities (work packages) required to complete a project in terms of scientific, legal, and regulatory requirements. They also include

- defined decision points, milestones, evaluations, etc.
- the interdependencies of these activities with respect to technical, scientific, ethical requirements, or as internally defined.
- the standard duration estimates for all work packages.
- the organizational unit responsible for the work package.
- definition of the output of each work package.

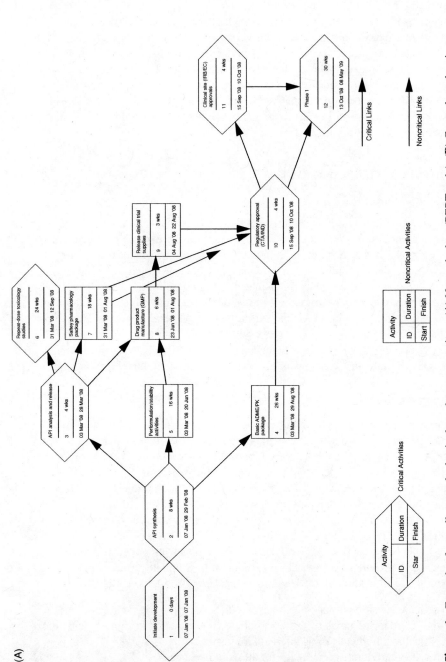

Figure 4 Example of a small network plan in three data presentations: (**A**) Network chart (PERT style). (**B**) Gantt chart showing critical and noncritical activities. (**C**) Table showing calendar dates and buffer lengths (prepared using Microsoft Project®). *Abbreviations*: API, active pharmaceutical ingredient; ADME; PK; GMP; CTA; IND; IRB; EC, ethics committee.

(B)

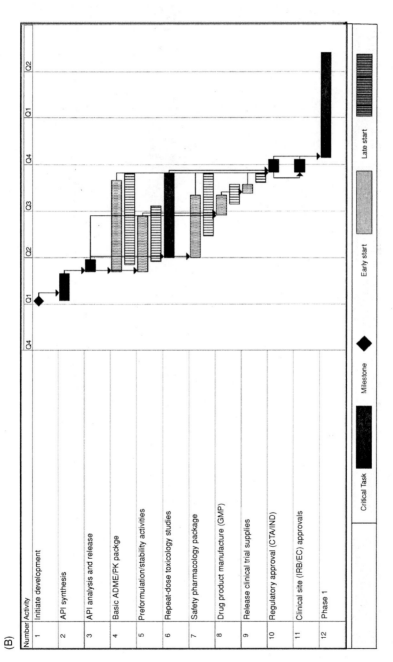

Figure 4 *(cont.)*

(C)

Number	Activity	Duration	Start	Finish	Early Start	Early Finish	Late Start	Late Finish	Buffer
1	Initiate development	0 wks	Mon 07/01/08	Mon 07/01/08	Mon 07/01/08	Mon 07/01/08	Mon 07/01/08	Mon 07/01/08	0 wks
2	API synthesis	8 wks	Mon 07/01/08	Fri 29/02/08	Mon 07/01/08	Fri 29/02/08	Mon 07/01/08	Fri 29/02/08	0 wks
3	API analysis and release	4 wks	Mon 03/03/08	Fri 28/03/08	Mon 03/03/08	Fri 28/03/08	Mon 03/03/08	Fri 28/03/08	0 wks
4	Basis ADME/PK package	26 wks	Mon 03/03/08	Fri 29/08/08	Mon 03/03/08	Fri 29/08/08	Mon 17/03/08	Fri 12/09/08	2 wks
5	Preformulation/stability activities	16 wks	Mon 03/03/08	Fri 20/06/08	Mon 03/03/08	Fri 20/06/08	Mon 24/03/08	Fri 11/07/08	3 wks
6	Repeat-dose toxicology studies	24 wks	Mon 31/03/08	Fri 12/09/08	Mon 31/03/08	Fri 12/09/08	Mon 31/03/08	Fri 12/09/08	0 wks
7	Safety pharmacology package	18 wks	Mon 31/03/08	Fri 01/08/08	Mon 31/03/08	Fri 01/08/08	Mon 12/05/08	Fri 12/09/08	6 wks
8	Drug product manufacture (GMP)	6 wks	Mon 23/06/08	Fri 01/08/08	Mon 23/06/08	Fri 01/08/08	Mon 14/07/08	Fri 22/08/08	3 wks
9	Release clinical trial supplies	3 wks	Mon 04/08/08	Fri 22/08/08	Mon 04/08/08	Fri 22/08/08	Mon 25/08/08	Fri 12/09/08	3 wks
10	Regulatory approval (CTA/IND)	4 wks	Mon 15/09/08	Fri 10/10/08	Mon 15/09/08	Fri 10/10/08	Mon 15/09/08	Fri 10/10/08	0 wks
11	Clinical site (IRB/EC) approvals	4 wks	Mon 15/09/08	Fri 10/10/08	Mon 15/09/08	Fri 10/10/08	Mon 15/09/08	Fri 10/10/08	0 wks
12	Phase 1	30 wks	Mon 13/10/08	Fri 08/05/09	Mon 13/10/08	Fri 08/05/09	Mon 13/10/08	Fri 08/05/09	0 wks

Figure 4 (*cont.*)

The computer planning software calculates an overall duration and shows the critical path as well as time buffers or float. All activities in individual project plans should relate to these standard work packages through a description term or number.

To be a reliable tool, the standard plan must be regularly updated by the designated personnel to comply with new regulatory and legal requirements and changed company procedures. Standard time estimates for experimental studies should reflect the time targets of the responsible departments for executing the task under standard conditions without abnormal resource constraints and unexpected problems. When available, benchmarking data from high-performing competitors should be used to set the standard durations.

The level of detail included within network and standard plans should be appropriate to capture the essential elements associated with the work package. Further breakdown is likely to be required within functions to ensure that overall project time lines are met within the network plan.

Information Systems

Requirements for Single Project Planning

When starting on a new project plan, the team lists tasks, defines work packages, determines predecessor/successor sequences, and asks for time duration estimates. The clearest way to present and discuss this information is the classical bar or Gantt chart. It is useful to document and organize it by using one of the many available project management softwares. This allows quick and easy changes, presentations in various levels of detail or in various timeframes, "what-if" scenarios of alternative ways to proceed, and clear presentation of the data.

The critical path of a project, typically, is evident without computer help; however, it is useful to see the early and late start dates of noncritical activities and to use this information for resource scheduling and management of expenditure. Many software packages allow entering original and revised plan dates for convenient tracking and preparation of progress reports.

For these reasons, the use of planning software for pharmaceutical development projects is recommended. The systems may be PC or server based. Some of the more frequently used systems are listed in Table 7.

Detailed information regarding the features, system requirements, and comparison between different products can easily be obtained via a Web search. Reviews and comparisons can also be found in a variety of computer publications (4).

The choice of a system will be governed by the scope and complexity required and by the infrastructure of the company; for example, the requirement of a major pharmaceutical company or clinical research organization will differ markedly to that of a "start-up" biotechnology company.

The advent of Enterprise Project Management (EPM) products offers planning, scheduling, resource management (including time recording), portfolio

Table 7   Project Planning and EPM Software

Product	Vendor
Multiuser EPM systems	
Microsoft EPM 2003 and 2007	
	Microsoft
ARTEMIS 7, 9000, and ArtemisViews	Artemis International Solutions
	Corporation (Versata Enterprises, Inc.)
Open Plan™	Deltek
Project Planner (P3®) and Primavera P6™	Primavera Systems, Inc.
OPX2	Planisware
Clarity™ Project and Portfolio Management	CA™ Clarity
Project Planner Server and Enterprise Editions	Smartworks
Single Project/Stand-alone systems	
Microsoft Project	
	Microsoft
Fast Track Schedule	AEC Software, Inc.
Micro Planner X-Pert	Micro Planning International
Project Scheduler PS8™	Sciforma Corporation
SureTrak® Project Manager	Primavera Systems, Inc.
Project Planner PE—Personal Edition	Smartworks
Open Workbench	Clarity Division, BSO (CA)

Abbreviation: EPM, Enterprise Project Management.

review, and risk analysis together with document handling capabilities within the same system. This is an evolving growth area leading to escalating levels of sophistication.

Multiproject Planning Systems

The different functional departments in an organization need an overview of their ongoing and planned activities to track and schedule resources.

The system requirements for multiproject management within departments are very different depending on the amount and complexity of data and geographical location. The EPM products enable ready access to relevant data both to the functional departments and the project manager.

The relative expense, IT support required, and level of functionality provided by these sophisticated systems limit their use to the larger organizations.

Management Information Systems

Senior management, investors, and potential development partners require top-level information on project plans, status, and progress. Typically, this is the level of milestones, general and specifically defined decision points, and time-critical activities. These data can be readily shared through the EPM systems.

SUGGESTED FURTHER READING

Mathieu M. New Drug Development: A Regulatory Overview. Cambridge, Maryland, MA: Parexel International Corporation, 1990.
Spilker B. Multinational Pharmaceutical Companies. Principles and Practices. 2nd edn. New York: Raven Press, 1994. Section III.

REFERENCES

1. Keyhani S, Diener-West M, Powe N. Are development times for pharmaceuticals increasing or decreasing? Health Aff 2006; 25 (Suppl 2):461–468.
2. Boyd RA, Lalonde RL. Nontraditional approaches to first-in-human studies to increase efficiency of drug development will microdose studies make a significant impact? Clin Pharmacol Ther 2007; 81:24–26.
3. Kola I, Landis J. Can the pharmaceutical industry reduce attrition rates? Nature Rev Drug Discov 2004; 3:711–715.
4. Project Manager Today. Software Tools Directory. Available at http://www.pmtoday.co.uk/content/en/toolsdirectory.aspx. Accessed on 2007.

4

Project Management of Chemical, Analytical, and Formulation Development

Dieter Krimmer

Rapid Pharma Development GmbH, Unteraegeri, Switzerland

INTRODUCTION

This chapter is about project-managing the closely related development disciplines of chemical, analytical, and formulation development. The chapter starts with a description of the key activities undertaken by each of these functions during development, registration, and product launch. Then the relationship of these activities, both within chemistry, manufacturing, and controls (CMC) and with other project team activities, is described from a project-planning perspective. The final section highlights CMC project management strategies that can be followed to achieve early market entry, to minimize the risks to the overall project, to ensure that the investments in work activities are triggered at the right time, and to ensure that a robust registration package is submitted that will convince the regulators that the sponsor company is in control of the drug substance and the drug product manufacturing processes.

OVERVIEW

The pharmaceutical industry has a reputation for the high quality of its products. A historical perspective helps to understand why the industry operates to demanding regulations in the manufacture of medicinal products. In 1937, the Massengill Company of America marketed a formulation of sulphanilamide dissolved in diethylene glycol. One hundred and seven children died after taking this medicine.

Between 1959 and 1962, it is estimated that 10,000 children were deformed as a result of their mothers taking thalidomide during early pregnancy. Legislation was enacted in both the United States of America and the United Kingdom requiring manufacturers to provide evidence of efficacy and safety before the marketing of a drug would be allowed. The assurance of the safety of the medicinal product rests upon knowing what it contains and that whatever it contains has been adequately evaluated in toxicology studies and clinical trials.

CMC comprises a major section in the regulatory dossier for marketing approval of a new drug. Central to the principle of control is the setting of a specification for the drug substance and the drug product. The specification itself requires that accurate, sensitive, and reproducible analytical methods be developed so that there can be confidence that whatever is present will be reliably detected and quantified. The release for use of the drug substance or the drug product is conducted against the specification. Preclinical safety studies in animals are conducted to define the margin of safety of the drug substance batch that is administered. The impurity profile of the batches used in the animal safety studies is carefully monitored. The animal studies, in essence, qualify that the defined amounts of the parent drug and the associated defined levels of impurity can be administered to humans with reasonable safety. The safety of such doses in humans is then evaluated in the clinical trials program. This information can be used to set acceptable levels of impurity in the drug substance or the drug product specification. The drug product must remain in specification for its shelf life, which might be three to five years for a tablet. Evidence is needed from stability trials that the specification will still be met in the storage conditions allowed within the proposed market label. The key CMC activities supporting the registration submission are performed to a demanding system of quality control known as Good Manufacturing Practice (GMP). This requires sponsors to be able to provide evidence that the manufacture of the drug product has been compliant with GMP requirements. An important safeguard is the separation of "powers" for the three elements namely manufacture, quality control, and quality assurance. Audits are conducted to check not just that GMP standard operating processes are in place at the manufacturing site but also that there is evidence of them having been followed. In addition to the audits commissioned by sponsors for contracted manufacturing, the FDA also visits manufacturing sites to satisfy themselves that appropriate quality standards are in place.

A number of important challenges emerge from the above that set the frame-work for the phases of CMC development for a new chemical entity entering preclinical development. Firstly, the route of synthesis that has been used to make small amounts of drug for the discovery group will need to be changed and optimized to supply development needs and also to supply the markets with the drug at minimized cost. Secondly, analytical methods will need to be established that are fit-for-purpose to enable a specification to be set. Thirdly, the "product" (what will be sold) will need to be developed. Formulation development studies will be initiated and stability studies will be conducted.

The compound supply will be time-critical because a number of development activities need to be sourced. Careful planning of the CMC work to support the development program is essential. Not only is there a need to maintain accurate logs of supply and demand but the allocation of batches to particular studies also needs careful review. Chapter 3 describes how planning is carried out at the project level and highlights some key steps in the drug substance, drug product, and analytical areas. In the following sections, the work of the CMC team will be described in more detail. This will lead into a description of project management of CMC from strategic and operational perspectives.

Chemical Development

The chemical development group is tasked with discovering a robust (reliable) and viable (in terms of cost, environmental impact, and safety) commercial process for the synthesis of the drug substance on a manufacturing scale and to transfer this technology to the site of manufacture. It is worth noting at this point that earlier medicinal chemistry has had very different objectives namely to discover a chemical that interacts with a biological system with the effect of modifying a disease state. These different objectives mean that the synthetic route of the medicinal chemist generally is not optimized and indeed intermediates may have been chosen so as to be easily converted to related structures to define the structure–activity relationship for the target receptor. With the focus now on a selected development molecule, route optimization can proceed.

There are three main phases to the work carried out in chemical development:

- Rapid establishment of a viable supply route to fund activities of other development groups; 1 to 10 kg quantities may be required depending on the drug potency
- Discovery of the best synthetic sequence, i.e., identifying the key intermediates
- Development of the best synthetic sequence into a safe, economic primary manufacturing process

To achieve these objectives, a thorough understanding of the chemistry involved in each step of the synthesis is required.

Supply Route

The first task is to establish a viable route of supply capable of preparing the required quantities of drug substance for early development needs such as one-month toxicology, phase 1 clinical studies and formulation development. Typically, it should be possible to prepare 1 to 10 kg of drug substance in a timely manner by the chosen route. The first step is to evaluate the medicinal chemistry route and determine what features render the route difficult to operate on a larger scale (e.g., highly toxic reagents, reagents not obtainable on a large scale, multiple chromatographic purifications). Modifications to the medicinal chemistry route would be quickly established in the laboratory and, in some cases, a completely new approach would be adopted prior to the scale-up in the laboratory or pilot plant.

Best Route

After a route of supply is established, the discovery of the best synthetic route can be undertaken. This stage of work, carried out by chemists in chemical development, requires retro-synthetic analysis and the use of chemical literature and online databases to propose several "paper chemistry" routes to the desired drug substance. The routes are prioritized and evaluated in the laboratory and the most appropriate sequence (with regard to length of the sequence, reagent availability, environmental impact, and cost) is chosen and scaled up further in the laboratory and pilot plant. After successful demonstration, a suitable pilot-plant process for carrying out each stage of the chosen sequence is developed and optimized. This then becomes the final route of synthesis. It is important from a cost and regulatory viewpoint to establish the final synthetic route to supply major time-demanding development studies (i.e., two-year carcinogenicity studies, phase 3 clinical studies, etc.). Some further modification to the chemistry will still be possible provided that it does not significantly change the impurity profile of the drug substance. If it is commercially desirable to adopt new chemistry where the impurity profile is significantly altered, bridging toxicology will be required and this will have cost and time implications.

As the demand for drug substance continues to rise, more pilot-plant batches of the chosen sequence will come out. Experience with these pilot-plant batches will provide valuable data about the robustness of a process and highlight areas for further development and control of impurities.

If the drug substance has an optical center, then the separation and biological testing of each enantiomer will have generally been carried out in medicinal chemistry. Nowadays, development and marketing of racemates must be justified (e.g., the enantiomers are equipotent, racemization occurs very rapidly, etc.). If a single enantiomer is required then chiral chromatography of a diastereomeric derivative or classical resolution are common techniques to make the desired enantiomer available. A long-term enantiospecific route development would also be explored.

Final Manufacturing Process

Once the final synthetic sequence has been established, it will be developed into the final primary manufacturing process. In this stage of the work, carried out by chemists in chemical development, the best reagents, solvents, and conditions need to be established for each transformation in the final synthetic sequence. A deep understanding of the chemistry at each stage is required to enable a rational choice of conditions to be established. In addition, the minimization and control of impurities at each stage needs to be understood. The "boundary conditions" (i.e., the conditions within which the process is guaranteed to produce an acceptable quality product) at each stage are established during this phase of work. When the final process is developed, it is demonstrated on a pilot scale prior to transferring the technology to the manufacturing site. Many reaction conditions and reagents can be used on a pilot-plant scale with suitable engineering but each solution has an associated cost.

An important part of the work of chemical development is to consider the environmental impact of the waste streams. It is often possible to minimize the environmental impact by careful design of the final process. Part of the package of information required for the transfer of technology to a manufacturing site is the characterization of the waste streams.

Formulation Development

The formulation development program will be tailored according to the type of pharmaceutical form to be marketed. To illustrate the type of activities that commonly have to be undertaken in formulation development the text will focus upon the development of an oral-dose form for a chronic therapy drug. Some general comments are relevant on what will be "key deliverables" from the formulations group as the development proceeds.

- The drug will likely need to be formulated to enable it to be adequately orally absorbed in animals and in humans.
- Animal toxicology studies will often require a formulation of the drug that can be administered by oral gavage. In some studies, capsule formulations may be used in larger animals such as dogs.
- The phase 1 first–in-human study generally explores a wide range of doses starting with likely subtherapeutic doses, testing of six to eight dose levels of drug, in common. Simple formulations (drinking solution, simple capsule) are typically used supported by short-term stability data.
- Phase 2 studies, typically, will test three to four dose levels of the drug with the intent to identify the optimal dose to take forward to phase 3 clinical trial.
- The formulation to be tested in phase 3 efficacy trial should ideally be the formulation that was first introduced into the market. If there is a change in the formulation, evidence for bioequivalence between the phase 3 formulation and the one to be marketed will be required.
- To register the drug for the market, data will have to be submitted to regulatory agencies to support the shelf life of the product as it is described in the package insert. An adequate shelf life (at least two years) is commercially important for a chronic therapy drug.

The formulations group will structure their work program to meet these demands. Physicochemical characterization of the drug is usually conducted in the selection of the lead. Sometimes, a decision may be made to change the salt form to optimize some attribute (stability, solubility) at an early preclinical phase. Preformulation studies may assess a selection of simple types of formulation with capsules or tablets. Dissolution rate testing will define whether the drug is sufficiently rapidly released under pH test conditions mimicking those in the GI tract and whether there is acceptable variability. Since the optimum clinical dose is not known at the start of development, several capsule or tablet strengths may be made. These will be put on a stability trial, which includes stress testing at conditions of high humidity and temperature, to determine whether there may be problems in long-term storage. The results from these studies will influence decisions on the packaging that will be used (e.g., aluminum blister packs, if they show humidity sensitivity).

Analytical Development

The development of sensitive and reproducible analytical methods is central to the whole CMC program. This applies to the process of manufacture of the drug substance and to the formulated drug product. The measurement of the purity of the drug substance and the impurities and degradants will require the establishment of validated assays and the synthesis of reference standard. The scope of the work program is considerable. Long-term stability trials running over several years are required for the representative manufacturing batches that will be cited in the registration dossier.

Primary and Secondary Manufacturing

Primary manufacturing refers to the active pharmaceutical ingredient (API) manufacture and secondary manufacturing to the drug product manufacture. The drug product consists of the formulated tablet with a distinctive shape, color, and markings together with the primary packaging, which may be a blister pack, and secondary packaging, which may be a carton with a labeling that will have to meet the regulatory requirements.

In some companies, there are dedicated market entry plants that are designed to support production of the drug to volumes sufficient to support market entry. The concept is to switch primary manufacture potentially a couple of years after the product launch. In other companies, primary manufacture technology transfer from a pilot plant to the manufacturing site is prior to registration. This puts pressure on the chemical development to select the final route and transfer it to the manufacturing site so that the representative batches can be made. Regulatory agencies require that "representative batches" of the API and the drug product are made and the data pertaining to the quality of these runs are submitted in the new drug application (NDA) application. FDA approval for a new drug is given if the drug can be shown to be safe and effective for the conditions prescribed in the package insert and if it can be demonstrated that the methods, facilities, and controls used for its manufacture, processing, and testing are adequate to ensure and preserve its identity, strength, quality, and purity. GMP establishes principles and processes to ensure that there is verifiable evidence that required standards were achieved in production and quality control. GMP has a central importance to

CMC project management and also to all aspects of decision-making during the development, registration, and in-market phases.

CMC ACTIVITIES AND THE PHASES OF THE PROJECT

The description of the CMC activities given above gives a flavor of the scope of the work. However, it does not adequately convey the intensity of the interrelationships of the chemical, analytical, and formulation development groups. Probably it is impossible in diagrammatic depiction to get close to how it works in the real world. This is why the way the CMC team works together as a team is such a critical success factor. This topic will be revisited later. For now, it is valuable to walk through the phases of development to see how the "CMC threads" are interwoven to create the medicinal product and to explore the linkages to the broader project development plan. This will reveal some of the challenges and pressures that the CMC team works under and will serve as a preface to the following section, which will propose successful strategies for CMC management.

The main activities undertaken by the three CMC functions are summarized in Table 1 according to the phase of development. The nomination of a lead compound to enter preclinical development by the discovery group follows on from an extensive program in which the structure–activity relationship will have optimized to achieve a drug with high selectivity and adequate potency for a defined biological target. A package of work will have been completed that will have defined the basic physicochemical properties of the drug and a variety of in vitro and in vivo tests to screen out the undesirable absorption, distribution, metabolism and excretion (ADME) attributes. Basic mutagenicity tests will usually have been conducted. With the drug now in the preclinical development phase, the objective is to develop the data to be able to judge whether the candidate is fit-for-purpose to be tested in a first–in-human trial. The major challenges during this preclinical phase for the CMC team would include getting to grips with the route of synthesis to select the supply route since a number of in vivo studies will be conducted during this phase to evaluate the safety of the drug such as safety pharmacology studies and single- and repeat-dose (14- or 28-day) toxicology studies in two species. Therefore, it may be necessary to rapidly supply 5 to 10 kg of API, which in turn would supply the toxicology studies and the phase 1 first–in-human study. The API will be formulated to optimize its presentation to the GI tract so that adequate bioavailability and exposure is achieved. This may be quite challenging because toxicology studies are conducted to determine what adverse effects are seen in animals when much higher doses than the expected therapeutic doses are tested in order to identify a safety margin of exposure. As a result, high concentration of the drug will be used in the dosing vehicle and formulation approaches will be required to support the best presentation of the drug in these circumstances. In rodent toxicology studies, oral gavage of solutions and suspension are dosed. Larger nonrodent second species may be dosed with capsules. In preclinical development, there is a major

Table 1 Summary of CMC Activities by Phase

	Lead Optimization	Preclinical	Phase 1	Phase 2	Phase 3
Chemical development	File candidate nomination	Select method of synthesis	Establish synthesis	"Freeze" the synthesis	Transfer technology for API to manufacturing site
	Review syntheses	Source starting materials	Source starting materials	Select manufacturers of starting materials	Make 3 representative API batches at the manufacturing site
	Determine API physicochemical properties	Identify impurities and isomers	Confirm impurities and isomers (make them)	Make impurity and isomer reference standards	Prepare documentation for regulatory submissions
	Initiate small-scale supply (<100 g)	COGs V-1	COGs V-2	COGs V-3	
		Determine feasibility of synthesis	Scale up feasibility	Establish large-scale synthesis	
		Start synthesis of phase 1 drug	Start synthesis of phase 2 drug	Further ICH stability data on API	
			Obtain ICH stability data API		
Analytical development	Characterize the drug	Develop HPLC methods for API and impurities	Establish HPLC methods for API and impurities and isomers	"Freeze" HPLC methods (API and impurities; if possible, also for isomers)	Transfer analytical methods to manufacture sites for API and drug product

Evaluate analytical methods	Develop HPLC method for the drug product	Establish HPLC for drug product	"Freeze" HPLC method for the drug product	Prepare analytical documentation for regulatory submissions
	Conduct prevalidation of HPLC method	Develop stability indicating HPLC method	Conduct validation of all analytical methods	
	Set first specification for API and drug product	Conduct validation of HPLC methods	Set final specifications for API and drug product	
	API: crystalline; polymorph	Set API and drug product specifications		
Formulation development	Develop formulations for phase 1	Develop formulations for phase 2 trials	Develop phase 3 formulations	Transfer technology for drug product to the launch site
Screen formulations for toxicology	Perform stability study in phase 1	Obtain ICH stability study for phase 2 formulation	Obtain ICH stability data for phase 3 formulation	Make 3 representative batches
	Make phase 1 supplies	Make phase 2 supplies	Make phase 3 supplies	

Abbreviations: API, active pharmaceutical ingredient; COG, cost of goods (sold); ICH, international conference on harmonisation; HPLC, high performance liquid chromatography.

push to establish analytical methods to test the purity of the API and identify impurities and degradants. Typically, the purity of the API at this stage is not as good as that which will be achieved at a later stage. It is important to qualify the drug substance being synthesized at this stage in the toxicology studies so that it can be dosed to volunteers albeit at much lower doses. Under the European Union Clinical Trial Directive, the investigational medicinal product must be manufactured to GMP if it is to be tested in phase 1 studies. There is often a need to do further physicochemical characterization work and, on some projects, a decision may be made to switch to new salt forms that offer particular advantages such as better solubility or stability.

During phase 1, which often takes about 10 to 15 months to complete, the chemical development will move from the initial "supply" route to the "best" route and a broad array of high performance liquid chromatography (HPLC) analytical methods will be put in place to measure impurities and degradants in the drug substance and in the clinical trial supplies. The clinical group will be establishing the protocols for the phase 2 clinical program and the project team will agree to the predicted dose range for phase 2. The formulation group works closely with the clinical group to ensure that clinical supplies match the trial needs. Placebo dose forms and the need to conduct blind studies may influence the supplies to be manufactured. The dose range to be studied in phase 2 may be quite wide (e.g., 20, 40, 80, 160 mg, etc.). Stability studies are needed to assure that the clinical supplies remain in specification under the conditions and duration of use. Stability studies will often have a matrix design that enables the stability data of the dose to be used (in this case, 20 and 160 mg) to support an assessment of the stability of the intermediate doses. If the tablets in the phase 2 studies are to be of the same size for all doses, it will require appropriate adjustment of the active-to-excipient ratio. The dissolution profiles of the different tablet strengths will need to be checked to ensure that release characteristics are affected. A cost of goods assessment will be made (current/anticipated). Supplies will be needed for the long-term toxicology studies such as the six-month rat and nine-month dog studies, which will enable extension of clinical dosing periods.

During phase 2, the experience gained with the "best" route of synthesis will enable the selection of the "final" route of synthesis, which is the route to be used to manufacture the phase 3 pivotal registration clinical trial supplies and the product to be launched into the market. The final route of synthesis is also used to supply the lifetime studies in rats and mice. International conference on harmonisation (ICH) stability studies will be initiated for the API and the tablet formulation. Cost of goods will be revisited. The clinical group will develop the protocols for the phase 3 trials. These trials will generally involve studies against the approved drugs. The comparator drug will need to be sourced and a strategy be decided for appropriate blinding of the study. Since the phase 3 trials will likely involve many sites and countries around the world and recruit potentially 1500 to 3000 patients who will be dosed for up to a year, a considerable effort will go into clinical trial supply manufacture, packaging, and labeling. The CMC team will prepare for regulatory exchanges such as the end of phase 2 meeting with

FDA to confirm that the phase 3 CMC plans are on target to provide an acceptable registration package.

In phase 3, the final route of synthesis is transferred to the API manufacturing site and the technology transfer for the tablet manufacturing process transferred to the product manufacturing site together with the transfer of the analytical methods. Both sites will need to have been audited and be GMP compliant. Representative batches of the drug substance and the drug product will be made. The manufactured drug substance and drug product will be put onto stability trial. One year of stability data is usually required at the time of the registration filing. The clinical dose for the lead indication will be known. The commercial group will provide input on tablet design and packaging. The CMC team will work to assemble the regulatory submission. A further assessment will be made of the cost of goods.

During the registration phase, ongoing stability studies will be reviewed to assess the likely viable product shelf life. Launch stocks will be manufactured to achieve adequate market entry support. The formulation development group often will be undertaking commercially driven life cycle management initiatives to refine the presentation. The chemical development will continue to explore ways to improve the API synthesis with a view to postlaunch cost-reduction initiatives.

CMC PROJECT MANAGEMENT STRATEGIES

The main challenges the CMC team faces can be broadly summarized as follows: to reduce time, to reduce risk, and to reduce cost. Actually, there is a significant interdependency between these objectives. For example, contingency actions to reduce risk need to be funded. Considering these three challenges is a good way of reviewing CMC strategies. The "right" CMC strategy clearly will, in many cases, be dependent on the type of the pharma company—what resources does it have in people, processes, and facilities. At one extreme are the top 10 pharma companies that have considerable in-house facilities, technologies, processes, and people who can be put behind priority projects. At the other extreme is a small biotech working in a virtual project team environment in which all work is outsourced and managed by consultants. The author has extensive working experience in both of these terrains.

Reducing Time to Market

In chapter 1, it was pointed out that development times were shortened during the 1990s probably because of the advances in the efficiency of execution of clinical and more rapid issue of clinical reports. This has put pressure on the CMC team to "keep up" and to avoid being the group that is rate-determining to the filing of the dossier. It is clear that from the moment a drug is progressed to the preclinical development, the CMC team is multitasking driven by immediate supply and demand while also needing to cover the long-term development needs. Some basic questions involved are: What activities lie on the CMC critical path for a project? What is the shortest irreducible timeline for CMC activities? What activities potentially can be stripped out? A simple answer is to say that it all depends on the project. However, there are activities and "blocks of activities" that are always there in the CMC plan and some activities that are not. For example, the manufacture of the representative batches of the drug substance and drug product and the initiation and conduct of the related stability trials are core activities that will always be part of the CMC plan and often on or close to the critical path to dossier submission. In contrast, some companies can avoid what is often a time-consuming technology transfer step of transferring the final route of API manufacture from chemical development to manufacturing site if they have a market entry plant that can be used to support the launch and early market supply. Only a limited number of companies have such facilities available to them to save time in this way. However, other strategies are available to save time even without the "Rolls Royce" facilities of big pharma. Firstly, good strategic planning is needed to focus on the parts of the CMC cycle where real project timesavings can be gained. Getting to a decision point on the final route early is one example. There is a balance to be struck between a fit-for-purpose synthesis suitable for market launch and support and the desire to achieve a fully optimized synthesis with the attendant significant delay in getting there. If the final synthesis can be selected relatively early then the representative batches and the stability data can be provided earlier to the dossier and to the regulatory agencies. There will, in any case, be ongoing investments to improve the manufacturing process during the product life. It is important to fully explore during the discussion with regulatory agencies about what data is essential at the point of submission. In part, this will reflect the overall "sense" of the CMC data. If it is perfectly evident from the overall stability trials data that the product is stable and the product offers a promising advance in clinical benefit, regulatory agencies will generally not insist on a tick box "one-year stability data at submission." Put another way, smart companies work closely *with* the agencies to understand what is required beyond the book. Another general strategy that can save time is "development simplification." This might be described as the serial questions "Is it really needed?" and the supplementary "Is it really needed now?" People working in CMC will likely instantly empathize with this because they are acutely aware of the scale of additional burden of work that seemingly innocuous requests have on the already burdened groups. The demand of a rookie "marketer" to finesse the tablet for market entry must be challenged. For some projects, the marketing rationale may be there but for many others, particularly the innovative products, it is worse than a distraction—it is a wasteful use of talented resources already under heavy pressure on the main job. So, the "simplification question" needs to be serially asked throughout development—"Do you really need this?" "Nice to have or must have?" The project team has an important role to play here in helping the CMC team focus on the core program that is truly needed. In summary, faster times to market can be achieved by the CMC team. Time can be saved by a combination of specific strategies but more importantly by a consistent attitude that challenges additive work burdens, seeks always to simplify the tasks, and to reduce, whenever possible, the technology transfer steps.

Sourcing the Work: In-House and/or At Contract

Chapter 9 addresses the project management of contracted development. For small pharma companies, outplacement of CMC work is a necessity. The options are whether to try to run with a "one-stop shop" strategy or whether to opt for several contracts with contract manufacturing organizations for the workpieces. There are pros and cons with either strategy. A potential benefit of the one-stop shop strategy is to reduce the number of boundaries and interfaces. This is attractive, given the interrelated nature of the work in chemical, analytical, and formulation development. Potentially, since the CMC teams are working closely together, time may be saved, risk may be reduced, misunderstandings may be fewer, and the time taken to resolve issues may be shorter. However there are some disadvantages. A high level of dependency results from this strategy ("all the eggs in one basket") and the negotiating flexibility is likely eroded. Another approach would be to contract chemical development to one company, analytical development to another, and formulation development to another with separate contracts also for manufacture of the drug substance and drug product. This type of contracting strategy is common in the industry. The coordination of the CMC activities undertaken this way requires active management. There are hybrid solutions. For example, the placement of chemical development with one company can make sense but there is a dependency issue. Strategically, it is important to have a second manufacturer to reduce risk and to support price negotiation. Given the very close interrelationship of the chemical development work with the development of analytical methods, the placement of both these activities with one company is sensible if the company has a strong analytical group. When the final route has been selected and run and the process has been reported, batches of API can be contracted to a second API manufacturer.

Central Laboratories

If analytical work is contracted out to a number of analytical companies during development, it is vital that the work is very carefully coordinated. Transfer of assay methods from one laboratory to another laboratory quite often results in problems of reproducibility with different instruments. This can create significant confusion to the ongoing CMC development program and has led some to opt for a central laboratory strategy.

Cost Management and the Tendering Process

It is essential that the sponsor follows a clear process in the selection of contractors and in the award of a contract. The process requires that an adequate technical briefing document is prepared that describes the sponsor's expectations and is specific in terms of the deliverables, the specification of the deliverables, and the timeline for delivery. Clearly due to the nature of the work, CMC activities do not always go according to plan. Therefore, the contract should anticipate this and include provision for how deviations to plan will be addressed with additional work approval and a costing structure to enable adequate financial control. Decision on award of contracts should be taken by the biotech management team on the recommendation of the expert consultant and endorsement of the project team. The decision will likely be influenced by price but other factors such as perceived competence, track history, and speed of delivery usually are highly important.

Quality Assurance and Expert Consultants

While a small biotech of necessity must contract out CMC activities, ultimately as the sponsor it is responsible to ensure that the manufacturing work is carried out in compliance with government regulatory requirements. Therefore, it is essential that the biotech retains the services of expert consultants with a deep industry experience to advise the company on strategic and operational issues. The scope of the consultant responsibility will include advising in the creation of the CMC plan, selecting and shortlisting the preferred providers, drafting the technical briefing document, reviewing contractor bids, and working with the sponsor contract and business staff on the contract for the chosen contractor. Beyond this, the consultant will actively manage the relationship with the contractor and update the sponsor at regular project team meetings. The consultant group should include a qualified person able to visit and audit contractors before the award of contract and, as appropriate, during the period of the contract.

Regulatory Interfaces

Ultimately, the regulatory authorities decide whether the product gets to the market and the CMC dossier is a key part of their assessment. It is vitally important that a clear understanding is achieved during the development regarding what potential issues the regulator may have with the CMC program and what the first registration file needs to contain. Important opportunities to interact with the FDA are at the pre-IND stage and at the end of phase 2 meeting. In Europe, scientific advice and formal consultation meetings are available to the sponsor. As highlighted above, it is possible that the regulator shows some flexibility in the data required in the initial NDA dossier, if justified by the overall "sense" of the CMC package, and companies should explore this.

Running the CMC Team

The CMC subteam is a part of the whole core project team (Fig. 1). In the project team meetings, the CMC leader and the subpart leaders (analytics, chemistry, and galenics) should participate. The technical team has interfaces with many groups (Fig. 2). The CMC team recruits its members from the different departments of pharmaceutical companies and/or from contract manufacturing organizations and/or from consultant agencies.

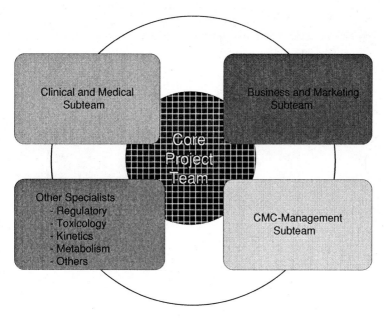

Figure 1

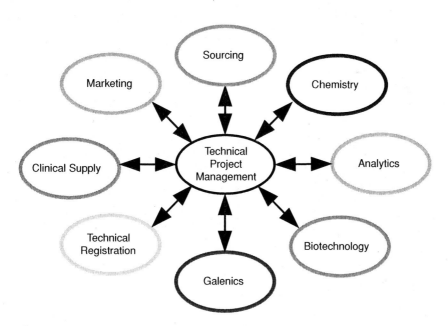

Figure 2

The CMC team should have regular meetings (weekly). In the meetings, all items must be discussed. Each member of the CMC team must bring in the issues for their departments. The meeting should be structured and should have a defined agenda:

- Minutes of the last meeting
- Project plan (updated)
- Sourcing
- Chemistry
- Biochemistry (if needed)
- Galenics
- Analytics
- Clinical supply
- Regulatory

The CMC team leader reports to the project leader and

- provides weekly updates,
- highlights scheduling issues on the critical path, and
- recommends solutions to the project team.

The members of the CMC team discuss all activities with their departments and make sure that the full expertise within the function is used to help resolve the technical issues of the project.

COST OF GOODS ESTIMATION

Cost of goods is monitored throughout the development process. Typically, the cost of making the drug substance is reduced dramatically during development as the synthetic route is optimized and yields get improved. Investment in route optimization continues after the product has been launched. Drug pricing for new drugs is generally not dictated by manufacturing costs but are driven more by the need to realize a return on the overall investment in R&D and the company costs in marketing the medicine. The situation changes dramatically when the drug goes generic and manufacturing costs become critical to pricing.

Figure 3 illustrates cost reductions for two principal routes and how to calculate which route is more cost effective. The author uses a system called cost evaluation system (CES), a sophisticated software based on an Access database to generate two products:

- Visualized process flow with a material balance adapted to the need of the customer (Example 1)
- Detailed cost calculation visualized in Excel sheets (Example 2)

To perform cost calculations, the customer has to enter only the defined master data and the material consumption in preprepared forms. These data can easily be modified, added, or deleted.

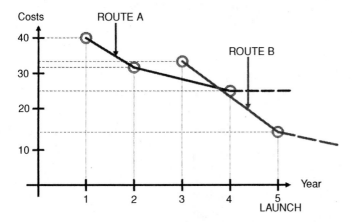

Figure 3   Cost of Goods and route comparison.

The key benefit arises from the speed with which calculations of complex processes can be set up and also modified. The evaluation of complex calculations can be assessed interactively (from several different sites).

Cost calculations using Excel sheets require changes of cell formulas for a lot of fields. CES was programed to be user friendly and can be used by pharmaceutical production people for budgeting or process optimization. In the development phase, it is an important tool for the project manager to calculate different scenarios for costing trends in the future or to evaluate key materials with different cost offers.

CES provides quick and accurate answers to specific questions about manufacturing costs. The key benefits of CES are that it

- is available at an affordable price,
- provides fast cost analysis of many possible manufacturing scenarios,
- requires minimal data input, and
- enables sensitivity analysis of cost drivers.

Some examples of the use of CES in estimation of costs of goods are shown below.

Example 1: "Flow Sheet" of a Process.
Example 2: Detailed Cost Calculation Visualized in Excel sheets
Example 3: Calculation for an APL

- Price of 1 kg API = €30,000 at phase 1
- 100 g API were produced on the laboratory scale
- Our calculation/estimation:
  - 100,000 kg API per year
  - 1 kg API = €750

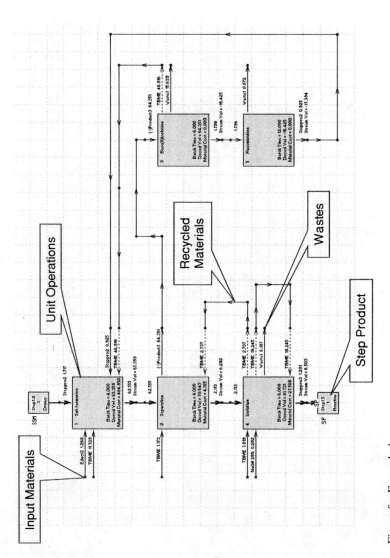

Figure for Example 1

SYNTHESIS YIELDS

PRODUCTION BLOCK UAT1 Chemicals:1
SIMULATION UAT1 Sim1

StartingPC1	200.00 kg/kmol	1.67 kg/kg step product	2.38 kg/kg end product	Through yield 23.96%
	Step Step 1.1 yield			
	89.00%			
Steppro1	150.00 kg/kmol	0.83 kg/kg step product	1.43 kg/kg end product	
	Step Step1.2 yield			
	75.00%			
Steppro2	240.00 kg/kmol	1.33 kg/kg step product	1.72 kg/kg end product	
	Step Step1.3 yield			
	75.18%			
Steppro3	240.00 kg/kmol	0.84 kg/kg step product	1.29 kg/kg end product	
	Step Step1.5 yield			
	81.31%			
Steppro5	350.00 kg/kmol	1.53 kg/kg step product	1.53 kg/kg end product	
	Step Step1.6 yield			
	65.33%			
Steppro6	350.00 kg/kmol			

PRODUCTION COMPARISON

Comment: (The Through Operating Costs figure is over all the steps in one production block.)

				COSTS ($F/kg)			
Simulation	Campaign mass kg	Yield %	Material	Operating	Fixed	Total	Through Operating

PRODUCTION BLOCK Chemicals:1
STEP Step5
ChemSim | 1006 | 782 | 2,068.27 | 0.00 | 0.00 | 2,068.27 | 30.13

PRODUCTION BLOCK Chemicals:1
STEP Step5
ChemSim | 1531 | 81 | 1,291.80 | 0.00 | 0.00 | 1,291.80 | 30.13

RAW MATERIAL COST SIMULATION

PRODUCTION BLOCK Chemicals:1
STEP Step2
SIMULATION ChemSim

Total cost of materials   469.70 $F/kg product
Simulated cost of materials   528.03 $F/kg product

Note:

Comment:

COMPONENT	ACTUAL PRICE	SIMULATED PRICE	
Ethanol	1.20	5.00	$F/kg

UNIT OPERATION VOLUME FACTORS

PRODUCTION BLOCK UAT1 Chemicals:1
STEP Step1.3

Comment:

UNIT OPERATION		VOLUME FACTORS (l)		
Name	Number	Stream volume	Dosed volume	Dosed volume (OR)
Salt formation	1	3711.26	3711.26	0.00
Isolation	4	969.24	2969.57	0.00
Separation	2	357.26	4011.26	0.00
Base/B(solation	3	-932.67	3954.00	0.00
Racemization	5	-987.67	-932.67	0.00

Figure for Example 2

- Real price after five years:
  - ○ 1 kg API = €700

    Example 4: Calculation for a Drug Product

- Manufacturing of tablets
- Contractor's offer for the price of the tablets:
  - ○ 1000 tablets = US $75
- Our calculation/estimation:
  - ○ 1000 tablets = US $55
  - ○ Without markup
- Real price after negotiation:
  - ○ 1000 tablets = US $60

5

Project Management in Exclusive Synthesis[a]

Lukas M. J. von Hippel

AllessaChemie GmbH, Frankfurt am Main, Germany

INTRODUCTION

In the preface to the first edition of this book, Tony Kennedy wrote: "The audience for this book will most likely include those in drug development and project management, as well as pharmaceutical industry consultants and project managers in other industries, for example, chemical and food." He was absolutely right. Therefore, it was logical that a manager from a chemical company was asked to contribute to the second edition of this book. It also reflects the increasingly important interaction between pharmaceutical and chemical companies and the resulting challenges for the project managers in both industries. In the following chapter, the chemical industry's view of pharmaceutical projects will be described and some of the key success factors for projects will be discussed.

CONTRIBUTION OF CHEMICAL SUPPLIERS TO A PROJECT'S SUCCESS

Once a drug candidate is found, apart from the pharmacological development the chemical development must also start. The focus of a medicinal chemist's work is to identify possible new drug candidates. The later production is not his concern, rather information about effects of substances is most important to him. However,

---

[a] This work is dedicated to the memory of Dr. Rolf Hoffmann, one of the best partners for development projects I ever had. Rolf died too early on May 9, 2005.

having identified a potential drug candidate, the rules of the game change: More material will be needed for the different development stages; even when the total amount of material needed is still only very small, eventual production on tons scale has to be in the mind of the chemists involved. The chemical process should be at least similar to the later commercial process. This is because any by-products present will have to be studied as well, which will later lead to the accepted impurity profile of the drug substance.

The chemical research organization in charge will have to develop a chemical process that can be scaled up. At the same time, it has to be balanced with how much work it is reasonable to invest at a given time of a project's life. Knowing that the majority of projects will die during development, it would be overkill and a waste of money to develop a process and make it robust right at the beginning of development. To decide about the time and money spent on a project at a given development stage is therefore important and needs good communication and understanding between the development partners.

Twenty years ago, most pharmaceutical companies had their own resources for upscaling in-house while the external market was used for the supply of more or less standardized intermediates. Slowly but surely, some companies decided to use external expertise for further development work as well. This was the time when the custom manufacturing business became more important. Later, the chemical research organizations also evolved and often specialized in the preparation of smaller volumes. At the same time, new business models started to change the pharmaceutical innovation path, allowing spin-offs and virtual companies to attract funding to develop new candidates. Venture capital became increasingly relevant for the development for new drugs from newly founded companies, often based on just a single project and venture capital. The service these companies required differed from the service bigger companies needed. Not only the development of a given chemical product but also the development of the analytical methods, registration according to the applicable laws, and so on are all services now frequently requested.

With the development of this dedicated service sector, the pharmaceutical companies gained access to a broad variety of chemical and related services, allowing them to use the skills of more individuals than they could ever have sustained in-house. By combining the skills of different companies and consultants, there is the potential to speed up the development times and to make the best of limited patent lifetimes. There is a visible trend that more and more companies now understand the logic of the service model and develop suppliers to be their development partners. For project managers, this means a new challenge, since fresh ways of project management must be developed.

INTERACTION WITH SUPPLIERS

The segment of the chemical industry focusing on pharmaceutical companies is indeed a service industry. Customer orientation is a must. Only when a customer's project is successful can the supplier be successful as well. The interdependence of customer and supplier in this project business is enormous, but both have the same ultimate interest—to make the project happen.

The reasons to choose an external partner for intermediates or the active pharmaceutical ingredient (API) are often simple. Not every company in the world can offer all types of equipment or every form of chemistry. Therefore, some companies are specialized in particular classes of chemistry or in the handling of special classes of substances. Looking at the market place, there are only a limited number of companies on a global scale offering more or less all types of reactions ranging from small to commercial scale. Only these companies have a chance to supply total "solutions to customers" using a broad portfolio of chemical skills and equipment. Other companies have more of a niche player character, adding value at a special step in the synthesis or in a certain phase of the project.

Pharmaceutical industry projects are complex. At the customer and at the supplier level, various functions have to be combined to form a powerful project team.

From a project's perspective, Figure 1 shows a network in interaction with a customer. There are different functions on both sides, often mirrored in the two cooperating companies. The small black arrows show the intracompany interactions, while the broader, gray-filled arrows show typical external interactions between companies. For the chemical supplier, the customer is often represented by a person in procurement, in other cases directly by the project leader or somebody else working in R&D. Depending on the size of the company and the project, the coordination of the different functions may be done by just one person (or perhaps by a team) at the pharmaceutical company, and the same is usually true at the supplier company. This person has the role to coordinate all internal functions with respect to the external supplier. This person may have several functions simultaneously, such as those of project manager and chemist or project manager and marketing manager. Different companies have developed different strategies to coordinate the externally driven activities, but there is a general trend visible: In most big pharma companies, the procurement function is also responsible for the first external contact. This person will also arrange technical meetings involving all the other necessary functions. In smaller companies, this role might be taken by somebody in project management, but this person must also handle the internal coordination.

In the chemical company, the first and main face to the customer will usually be the responsible person in marketing. This person will interact with the customer and coordinate all internal functions and communications to ensure the project's success. The coordination of all relevant functions and the project management often belongs to that person in marketing simply because this person has the most up-to-date and best knowledge of the customer's status of the project. There are also organizations where the project management function belongs to the responsible person in R&D, following the logic that only this person can coordinate all internal functions effectively because he/she knows best the status

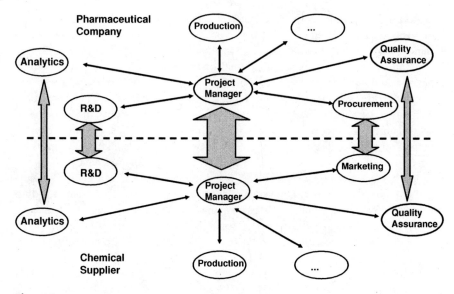

Figure 1

of the internal development work. Whichever structure is chosen, it is key that the two people can work together efficiently to make sure the customer's requirements are met in order to provide the desired material

- on time,
- in full,
- in spec,
- with all the relevant documentation and the regulatory support, and
- at a reasonable price.

These technical challenges take on human relations dimensions more or less immediately. In the past, researchers from different disciplines tried to understand why some projects were a success, while others failed. One of the key lessons learnt has been that the biggest part of human behavior is still driven and controlled by emotions. Even well-trained industrial employees are human beings and therefore the interaction with suppliers is also influenced by so-called soft factors. Some organizations even develop protocols to minimize the human element: Suppliers are compared and ranked according to given criteria. These criteria may be hard factors such as technologies, capacity, and performance, but may also contain soft factors, for example, credibility, communication, and responsiveness. It will be interesting to see how this model develops over the next few years; no matter how these models develop, they cannot avoid the human touch and the way interactions happen. From the project managers' perspective, they always have to make sure that human relations are in their focus and that they seek to understand the motivators of each and every member of their teams. This is not just a specialty of pharmaceutical projects and their management, but is also of a more general interest. Therefore, a good project manager will work to develop strong working relations with his/her project team and the team of his/her supplier or customer.

To be efficient, it is vital that the two people understand each other and also understand the way the different companies work and how decisions are prepared and made. It is important not only to get the people motivated but also to give them all the information they need to do the job properly and to stay motivated. When the success of a project is analyzed, it is astounding how often the real key success factor is the relationship between individuals and the trust they have in each other. Therefore, before we start with the first project, we must firstly try to build up a relationship with the counterpart in our client's organization. For us, this is the key factor for later success. To build this trust, we discuss openly and frequently and share information as well. Over the years, the understanding of the different organizations develops and the relationship improves. This relationship building may take time, even if legal formalities like confidentiality agreements are handled quickly and the wording is immediately understood by both sides.

BUSINESS CULTURE AND ETHICS

Working with external partners also requires that different company cultures work together. Not every company has the same ethos, quite apart from the fact that different cultures can clash and there might be some different expectations on both sides, for example, the interpretation of confidentiality or of the value of intellectual property. The concept of a "long partnership" may differ from company to company; it may not necessarily be part of a company's (or country's) culture but of the business ethics and what is convention.

National cultural behaviors have to be taken into account as well. The opportunities of a globalized world are closely connected to the risks. Therefore, the understanding of business ethics and the way different cultures do business is crucial. Members of international companies may be aware of the different interpretations of simple words and the trouble they might cause among colleagues, but this is also true for the interaction between companies. It does not mean that such interactions cannot add value, but it should be clearly understood that dealing on an international basis is always challenging. People who like to do it will develop with the years an understanding of the differences and will learn how to deal with it. There have been some great investigations about cultural differences between countries and people, one of the pioneers being Geert Hofstede who developed the so-called "cultural dimensions" and the tools to measure them. The easiest access to his findings is the Internet, but for a deeper understanding, his books are even better (1–5).

Confidentiality of projects is a must for the pharmaceutical industry. The structure of a new API or even of a key intermediate is often the most valuable information and has to be protected. To understand the importance of this is extremely important. Sometimes even the business relation between a sponsor and a supplier may be protected information as well, for example, when a small company is in negotiations for venture capital and wants to raise funds by having a big company as supplier for the API or the formulated drug in the background. In this case, even the name of the supplier will add value to the sponsor's project and this information must therefore be protected as well. Typically, all information that is more or less directly related to the project—from the perspective of the pharmaceutical company—has to be protected and, therefore, the supplier must do so.

The confidential information also includes the application fields of the new drug, the status of the clinical trials, chemical, pharmacological, or toxicological information, analytical methods, reference materials, impurities, and, of course, the project timeline and later commercial expectations. This list is not comprehensive, and there will always be more information in a project that the pharmaceutical company wants to keep secret. However, for the supplier, or better the development partner, it is very important to have information about the overall situation of the project. This helps to understand what actions should be taken and how to support the project in the best way. Supporting a project may mean sometimes to just stop the development work altogether to avoid adding further costs, but even then the picture should be clear for all the parties working together.

Sometimes, inconsistencies in the sponsor's organization become visible: From the project's perspective, all this information has to be kept secret, but other parts of the organization might have to use this information for other purposes to make it public. The project manager of a pharmaceutical company might like to keep everything secret, but the investor relations manager might, for other reasons, like to bring the pipeline, the status of a given project, and the future commercial potential including production volumes into the public domain. In particular, the later commercial expectations are often part of the discussions with analysts, and more and more companies tend to publish project data on their company Web pages, making them public. Therefore, it can be hard to judge as to what should be subject to confidentiality. In general, reliable partners will keep everything secret, even the name of the companies they cooperate with. Big companies might be seen to work with almost all organizations on a global scale, smaller companies might have some restrictions due to limited resources in marketing as well as in R&D and in production. Big players might be in a position to cover the majority of requested technologies, while smaller companies might play a role in niche technologies. However, a reliable partner will always keep confidentiality. Without written permission, he/she will never use customers' or project information for an advertisement or differentiation strategy.

On the other hand, the chemical supplier will also have intellectual property he/she wants to protect. The supplier's organization has special capabilities that make it well suited for the project. The supplier's interest will always be to have the freedom to use its technologies for other companies as well. After all, the business model is to serve the pharmaceutical industry in general and to offer services to the companies requiring them—as a full package or just parts of it.

This leads to a wider area of concern between the two parties as how to deal with intellectual property and how to protect it. In recent years, the industry has witnessed different routes of development into extreme positions: Some pharma companies have tried to secure all intellectual property not only on a project's basis but also the general technology background of their supplier. The acceptance of this position would usually have destroyed the supplier's business basis within a short time and therefore has not been generally acceptable. This position can also damage the basis of the interaction between companies, making it hard to rebuild a working relationship based on trust.

This leads to the key finding: Confidentiality—besides all legislative implications—is a part of business ethics and a confidentiality agreement is, first of all, only paper and a statement of how the partners intend to act. In some cases, the paper may not even provide an adequate basis for troubleshooting. In the past, some pharma companies intentionally tried to keep their supplier poorly informed, only providing some information on the overall status of the project. This led to the case that the development partner did not always correctly understand the real requirements for the project work. In some cases, the projects slowed down because the urgency for action was never properly appreciated, while in other cases the development partner acted too quickly and invested too many resources. Even if these examples are rare, the fact that they exist shows there is room for improvement.

Therefore, the selection of the development partner and the trust between the parties will be the most important ingredient for a later project's success. All people working for a long time in project management will agree that trust is a basic requirement for a project's success. If the partner is selected as a compromise choice, and is therefore not the most trusted one, the chances for the project to fail are extremely high. And vice versa, analyzing the best and most successful projects has led to the conclusion that the successful projects were characterized by a high level of mutual trust and understanding as well as recognition of the needs of both parties.

COMMUNICATION

The success of most big comedians results from playing with misunderstandings. Remember Laurel and Hardy? The two gentlemen always want to be kind, try to live with the rest of the world in peace, but fail to communicate in a proper way. So, at the end of the story, everything is in a mess and the spectator is amused. Or take the black comedy "War of the Roses": The inability of the couple to talk to each other and to keep communication going leads directly to the final catastrophe. Everybody also knows examples from their own experience. It is the reason why some jokes work: Take the joke of a man driving his car. The police stop him and he seems to be drunk. So the officer asks him to take an alcohol test. The driver answers, obviously delighted, "Certainly, officer, in which pub do you want to start?"

In most cases, misunderstanding does not happen because people want to be evil or want to destroy relationships or goods. It just happens because of a lack of communication or the misinterpretation of given information. So, one of the challenges for project management has been described and this challenge grows in times of globalization and at a time of complex projects involving specialists from different companies. A project manager needs to remember every day that communication is key. Communication is not only necessary to inform people, but also to keep them motivated, to make sure that they work in the same direction and that they have the same picture of the project status and the actions to be undertaken. Pictures can be a tremendous help to support communication and that is exactly the reason why project managers try to visualize as much as possible, for example, by drawing a project timeline, searching for the critical path, defining work packages with objectives, and so on. However, it does not mean that everybody has understood what is expected and that it is agreed: The project manager, therefore, has to anticipate:

- Spoken does not mean heard.
- Heard does not mean understood.
- Understood does not mean accepted.
- Accepted does not mean memorized.

So after every meeting and between meetings, the project manager must work hard to keep the communication going and to understand what might go wrong and what actions might be necessary to keep all people on track. If this work is not invested, the project might be trapped between different interpretations of what was discussed or shown. As a result, in the worst case, different prioritization of actions may happen in the different subteams. Depending on different information status the project team members have, the actions taken may differ as well. Therefore, the project manager has to frequently check the understanding of the team members to make sure that heard became understood and remained memorized. This is a hard job and, in particular, scientists coming from natural sciences tend to ignore it. So please stay aware of the really challenging fact that communication is more important than you ever dreamt and have fun with your next Laurel and Hardy film.

THE RIGHT PARTNER

Not every company can be the best partner for a given project. On a global basis, more than 1000 different companies claim to have the right chemical skills, the best trained people, and the highest innovation. Out of these, several hundred companies claim to have the best project management skills, to be open, honest, reliable, to have best practices, to work to ISO 9001 and/or 14001, to have access to all necessary analytical equipment, and so on.

The brochures from different companies are often remarkably similar and it seems that the whole world is working in the same way, with the same solutions provided optimally for their customers' projects. Reality, unfortunately, often looks different. There are a lot of projects where the suppliers do not add value, where communication does not work, and where the project slows down. Several times, I have had the chance to have a look at some of these projects and also had the chance to analyze the failures, refocus the project, and to speed it up again. I made two general findings on issues that slowed projects down or even brought them close to death: miscommunication, including different expectations of what the project should achieve, and the wrong partner with regards to company culture.

Before a company answers the question regarding who the right partner might be, the project and its requirements should be defined as precisely as possible: There will be large differences between the potential partners and their differences will determine success or failure. The second step should be targeting the potential partner for the development. It might be the case that different companies are best suited for the initial or later stages. Typical steps might involve moving from preclinical phase into phase 1 and from phase 2 to phase 3, and during the development phase the need to synthesize by-products on larger scale for toxicologic studies or for analytical questions. Again, depending on the requirements, not every company might be the right partner to solve the problem.

On the other hand, not every project will fit into the competencies and the focus of a particular organization. Therefore, most companies have developed tools to assess projects quickly and to evaluate their potential. For both partners it is important to understand the project potential. One of the best selection criteria for a potential sponsor might be to find out how the supplier's organization deals with inquiries: A potential supplier should never try to enter a project where it is not convinced to add value to that specific project. Only when the supplier believes himself/herself to be the right partner should he/she invest resources otherwise decline. This will save time and money. So one of the selection criteria for a potential sponsor might be the way projects are assessed and declined by the supplier. A supplier can provide a valuable service to a potential customer by directing them to an alternative supplier better able to meet their short-term needs. This might be the minimum service such an organization could offer.

PROJECT CLASSES

Nowadays, it is fairly common to differentiate projects by their complexity. As the term suggests, "exclusive synthesis" means that most of the chemicals produced are generally manufactured on an exclusive basis. There is a one-to-one relationship between the customer and the producer and the product is only applicable to a specific project. When the project dies, the product will no longer be of any commercial value. Molecules with less-elaborate structures might have a chance to be utilized in different products as advanced intermediates, while some of still lower complexity might be used as basic starting materials.

In addition, there exist three distinct types of projects that differ on a more general basis, namely

- custom manufacturing projects,
- contract manufacturing projects, and
- toll manufacturing projects.

Custom manufacturing projects are projects where the customer typically has a molecule just emerging from research and perhaps a first idea of how to synthesize it but no more information. For such a project, usually no technical information is available, and therefore the only information to share might be the structure or a chemical abstracts service (CAS) number. It is part of the project partner's job to develop a synthetic route, including all the in-process controls required, and sometimes even to develop an analytical method for the final product. Both customer and supplier will work together to find a workable specification and to fulfill all requirements from the authorities. The full range of support is required and, ideally, all functions should be in-house at the selected partner's site.

The best partner for such a development will be a company able to offer the full range of technologies needed, including the strongest analytical support. To have these technologies available not only on paper but also in reality, such a company should have a minimum size. Without this critical mass, a company is unlikely to have the financial and organizational power to have all relevant analytical equipment in place and might not be the best partner in terms of broad access to creativity to offer best solutions to the customer's needs. This type of company might also have the power to have a worldwide network of suppliers for raw materials and the power to direct them. Such a company might also have most types of the production equipment in-house leading to high flexibility in terms of realizable processes.

On the other hand, such a company might also have its limitations. For high-throughput screening substances, just a few milligrams are needed, so these companies might not be the best choice. Instead, there are smaller companies available, typically headed by a chemist with strong experimental skills, that are able to make small amounts of products in a short time. To focus on such a type of synthetic work needs other skills than those for production-orientated processes.

Contract manufacturing means the customer will be in the position to share a more or less detailed process with his potential supplier. The information available right from the initial project evaluation is more specific and therefore the need to protect the customer's interests will be even higher. For both parties it is easier to understand whether the process will fit into the potential supplier's production equipment and how the commercial production will look. On the other hand, there will still be a lot of open questions about how to adapt the existing process to the supplier's equipment and how to run the campaigns best.

The creative part of route design in these cases is more limited, but frequently there are still a lot of questions to be answered and such projects are still demanding. The transfer of knowledge from one company to the other is particularly important, and again, the nature of the interaction between the companies determines the level of success.

Toll manufacturing is the last type of project. Here the project sponsor not only provides the detailed process but also some of the key raw materials. This will be very interesting for both parties in the event that special technologies are requested and both companies in combination can offer an advantage that they do not have independently. This is the most extreme level of cooperation at the other end of the scale: While custom manufacturing requires a spirit of invention, toll manufacturing takes advantage of special technologies and the availability to run them.

For the responsible project managers of the two companies, the job is again more difficult than in the case of pure contract manufacturing: Even more functions of the two companies have to work together and interact to make the project a full success. Depending of the regulatory status of the product—non-GMP [not following good manufacturing practices (GMP)], c-GMP [current GMP], registered intermediate, or API—the complexity grows. Only open communication and a permanent comparison of the expectations of the two development partners allows both parties to optimize and reach a level they could not achieve independently.

ORGANIZATIONAL CONSEQUENCES AND PORTFOLIO MANAGEMENT

A chemical company dealing with exclusive synthesis is typically almost overwhelmed with work and inquiries. To manage this permanent overload and to keep it workable is part of the management function of the organization. Having products produced on a campaign basis means also that the utilization of the plants and the equipment varies permanently and has to be managed as well. In addition, the different levels of project complexity and different levels of requirements have to be balanced all the time.

Figure 2 shows, in a general way, how such a project-driven organization might look. The whole process is driven by the project managers who have an exceptional role within the organization. These managers need the support of all the relevant functions, for example, R&D, production, procurement, and QA/QC (quality control). On a project basis, colleagues from these areas will report functionally to the project manager who is supervising the project and keeping an eye on the targets. In a multiclient and multiproject environment, the different project managers themselves need supervision to deal with shifting priorities and allocations of resources. This is necessary to balance all the different projects with the requirement to reach an optimized utilization of resources.

From a project portfolio perspective, a company has to develop tools to balance the different requirements and to work with the tasks of multiproject management. There are not too many examples of organizations working almost totally in a project structure: The most common example is the consulting industry: This type of service is clearly driven by projects alone and therefore these companies give most of the power to their project managers. The rest of the organization has to support the projects activities, and conflicts of interest have to be settled by a steering committee. Such a company structure, typically matrix organized,

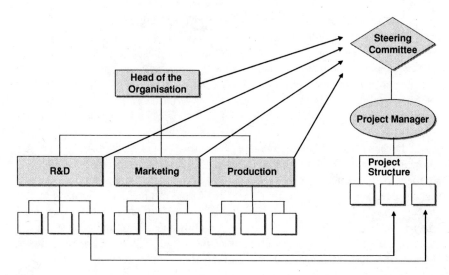

Figure 2

allows consulting companies to react quickly and to have the necessary specialists supporting the projects on an as-needed basis. All incentive systems for the
project managers reflect the quality of the projects delivered and give clear and
measurable targets. There are even companies that are totally driven by a traffic
light system where every project manager has to press the traffic light button for
his projects every week on Friday (Fig. 3).

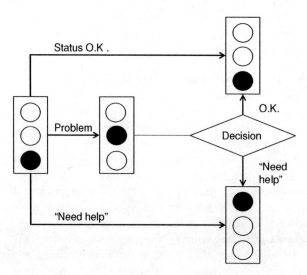

Figure 3

If the light is green, the organization accepts the status, and it is the project manager's duty to deliver the project on time, in budget, and in full. If the light is yellow, the project manager has the duty to press the button again on Tuesday in the following week. By then, the light has to be switched into red or green. If the light is green, it implies "all clear till next Friday". If the light is red, the board gets immediately informed and will take actions to get the project back on track. This example does not come out of the chemical or pharmaceutical industry nor from a consulting company but out of an industry driven by projects (unfortunately, I did not get permission to name the company and the business it is in). It is a highly efficient system to bring projects also in the top management's focus in an easy and self-explanatory way. This is an extreme position and shows how this particular company wants to manage projects and support the project managers. In this company, part of the company culture is that the board will take immediate action if a project is in danger.

The described organizational models can be transferred to a certain extent to the exclusive synthesis industry as well. Every inquiry received is a potential project, and the project will only end once the project dies for whatever reason or when a product reaches full commercialization and a long-term contract is signed. Even then, having production campaigns, every campaign will fulfill to a certain extent the character of a project. A characteristic feature of a project is that it has a start but also an end. Therefore, every project manager will keep in mind that the project's end has to be known and targeted right from the beginning.

In principle, there are two models available to organize the project management. In the first model, all project management activities will be driven by the person in marketing or business development, whereas in the second model the project manager is based in R&D. Both models have merits and limitations. In both cases, there are two key people in the internal project organization, the person in R&D and the person in marketing. They have to work very closely together and they have to reach a high level of understanding. There have also been organizations where the person in R&D also acted as marketing manager, but this model worked only in limited cases and, according to my knowledge, is no longer state of the art.

The assessment of a given project is clearly important and both parties, supplier and customer, share the same interest to find out whether the project will have a reasonable fit and whether the joint competencies of both companies can really add value to the project. This adding of value relates not only to the technological questions about the availability of somebody to make the product but also to timelines, availability of resources, and, of course, commercial expectations from both sides. This is often neglected and causes frustration later on. Therefore, most companies have developed tools to predict the likely cost of goods and can offer paper prices. A paper price is calculated from the chemistry performed only on paper, assuming yields and impurity levels, reaction times, analytical costs, development times, the more or less known prices for starting materials, costs for waste disposal, and logistics. If necessary, the cost for registration under

Example Research and Development, planning on Lab level

time (weeks)	1	2	3	4	5	6	7	8	9	10
Lab 1	project 1			project 3				free capacity		
	proj 2	project 4								
Lab 2	project 5									
	project 6								free capacity	
Lab 3	project 7									
	project 7			project 5						
Lab 4	project 7			project 3						
	project 1			free capacity						

Figure 4

chemical law will be included as well. However, both parties should have the same understanding regarding the paper price indication—it is just a guess and reality might differ, as all chemists know. Yields might drop dramatically for whatever reasons, material might not crystallize, by-products might challenge all purification methods, or the assumed reaction path might simply not work at all. On the other hand, the pharmaceutical industry has clear commercial expectations and a project has to pay off. If not, it will be stopped. There are also uncertainties relating to commercial expectations and potential—the bioavailability of a new drug is not known at the beginning, the indications may vary during the process of development as well, some of the by-products may later be identified as toxic, the formulation might be more expensive than expected, and so on. In fact, the real target costing may not be possible, only a target costing for the pill may be possible (after all, it is usually known what price the market will pay for a medicine). These risks have to be managed, which will be discussed later.

A supplier with multiple projects has to manage the workload of R&D, the utilization of production capacity in different plants, and the work for supporting functions like QA and analytics.

Figure 4 shows how the planning of resources can be done in a simple but efficient way. Balancing the workload and customer expectations of timelines to coordinate internal decision timelines with internal and external decision timelines is a daily challenge. The number of projects is typically higher than at a pharmaceutical company of comparable size. The logic behind this is simple: the API may contribute approximately 10% to the total turnover of a drug. Often the supplier is only allowed to supply advanced or key intermediates but not the whole API and in the case that they do supply the API, for risk management reasons there might be more than one supplier. So, the scope of the business available to a certain supplier is limited. Even for a blockbuster drug of more than one billion dollars annual turnover, the value of the API will only be in the range of $100 million. Assuming that the business is split between two suppliers, this means a two-digit million dollar deal for both of them. This is substantial business, but much less than the customer's turnover. When chemical and pharmaceutical companies have the same size, it clearly means that the supplier's organization needs more projects at a given time than the client. Clearly there is a need to develop well-organized instruments for multiproject management to handle this.

There will be some key criteria for supplier companies to decide about tendered projects. The first question will be about the technological fit and whether the supplier's organization has the potential to add value to the project. The next question will be about timelines to be kept. The project might have a perfect fit, but if the customer's expectations are not met there is no basis for collaboration. The timeline will comprise not only of the necessary laboratory availability but also the availability of production capacity. To balance the total project portfolio, other information will be requested to prepare the decision to go for a project or to decline it. This information will include the indication and phase of the project, the expected commercial volumes and, if available, a target price. Often it is easier to recalculate from a given target price the cost of goods and to come to a decision than to calculate from a paper price. The last topic is not surprisingly often the biggest point of discussion between companies but when the level of understanding between the companies, and therefore between individuals, is good, this hurdle will be passed easily.

As discussed above, the exclusive synthesis business is a project business and the project management organization has to manage the challenges of it. To do this smoothly, one of the key messages is to work in the future. When an organization works today on results that become relevant in the future, the surprises happening today will not cause trouble because the reaction time needed to deal with them has already been built in. This helps to minimize stress and pressure on people. At the same time, it necessitates discipline and a clear communication within the supplier and the customer organizations and also between the customer and supplier. It is obviously not easy to balance the challenges, but once it is done properly, the results achievable in a short time are astonishing. Only companies that have developed management skills to do this in an efficient way and then continue to improve will have a future in this business.

FLOW OF INFORMATION

Heinrich von Pierer, former CEO of Siemens, once said: "If only Siemens knew what Siemens knows. . ." The meaning behind was simply the fact that in bigger organizations the flow of information becomes more and more an issue and the availability of relevant information at the right time becomes increasingly difficult. That is why big organizations developed in the past numerous activities in knowledge management, often resulting in well-managed databases and research tools to make information available to those who need it. However, all this information can only be as good as the previously developed information that has been documented and catalogued. But the meaning of von Pierer's statement might even be deeper: It is not only the challenge to keep earlier generated knowledge accessible but also to keep information flowing across the organization and to make the right people aware that there is information available. Most people who have worked in a large organization can recall an occasion when the flow of information was not good and the lack of information caused not only repetition of work but also expensive actions of no additional value. On the other hand, not all information is relevant, and not everybody has to have knowledge about every detail at a given time. In a project world, it is up to the project manager to have the information and to decide about the necessity to share the information with others.

Having these examples in mind, the key question is how to avoid mistakes, especially in the interaction between companies. Not all data of a given project has to be shared with the supplier and vice versa. However, there are examples when a project died and nobody informed the supplier who was, of course, still working on the project. Only later, when the supplier was informed did the project end. Needless to say, this is not the best way to make friends. So, when a project generates important information, the person in charge should also think about the relevance of that information for others.

Typically, there is a gap between the different parts of a project. Chemical development often runs separately from the formulation work. Also, the structure of a development project reflects the different contributions that the subteams can make to the ultimate success. However, sometimes, life is not so simple that a chemical supplier can only contribute to chemical questions. By nature, a chemical supplier has to have analytical knowledge as well and so he might be able to support the analytical development. In addition, a chemical supplier might have plants operating under cGMP requirements, which would require that there are also people dealing with regulatory affairs. The input of these people might again help the overall project. Once an API is produced, it goes into formulation. The chemical industry does not often get access to the formulation data but there are cases where it could contribute to these questions too—solubility of an API might depend on the right salt, solvents might affect the later formulation, a special particle size distribution might support or hinder the drug release in a pill, and so on. Not every pharmaceutical company is prepared to take advantage of the interaction with a chemical supplier but there are more and more who are doing so. Again, to allow the chemical supplier to contribute to the project's success beyond the historical role needs a good understanding of the possible contribution and highly developed project management. In general, smaller companies tend to be more open to this way of cooperation but also increasingly big players understand the value of such an approach.

RISK MANAGEMENT

As readers will be aware, unfortunately nobody in the world is able to predict the success of a single project. Only in a portfolio of projects can a statistical approach be taken to predict the average survival chance of a project. For the pharmaceutical industry, therefore, the pipeline is one of the hottest topics for discussion with investors. The value of a company listed on the stock market depends not only on today's sales but also on the expectations of future business. And future business is, undoubtedly, represented by today's projects. For projects in development, there are average probabilities available for future success rates. There are estimates for future sales assuming prices, efficiency, market shares, and market developments.

Licensing of projects becomes an increasingly relevant business for all companies. The development of a new drug is a high-risk business and only a low percentage of all projects will ever pay off. In combination with increasing costs for development, companies are looking for opportunities to share the risk with others.

Besides the risk of a given project to fail due to unexpected clinical results, there are also risks from a purely chemical point of view: Not every chemical route can be scaled up, yields may drop by upscaling, impurities may cause problems, stability issues can arise, and so on. Newly identified intermediates may bring difficulties as well and may require special process designs unforeseeable events may happen every day in such surroundings. In addition, the pharmaceutical industry wants to have a safe supply situation including stable production conditions. However, in theory, a plane crash can cause the destruction of a production site within seconds. Even when these risks are low and the probability remote, they nevertheless remain. As a consequence, to keep the supply chain secure, single sourcing of special products or APIs from only one supplier is limited and often combined with a special stock-holding situation. More common is at least a dual-sourcing arrangement.

For the chemical supplier, this situation again increases the particular risk for a given project: The company is not only depending on the overall performance of a given project in the surrounding of a global pharmaceutical industry, but also on its own performance compared to competitors with exactly the same chemical structure. So, in addition to the normal project risk, the need increases because of competition to have the best and therefore most cost-efficient reaction path.

To turn the risk into opportunities is therefore the first task for project managers at the chemical supplier. With a proper evaluation of the chances and risks, and with an honest answer to the question whether his company can really add value to the customer's project, internal decisions are prepared to go ahead or to decline a project. And even the information that a project does not fit is valuable for the customer when given quickly. However, to come to a proper project assessment, the two parties must have a good understanding of each other. The openness of the potential sponsor is as important for the overall success of a project as the supplier's willingness to share information as well. Different expectations or understanding might cause irritation to one and might cause frustration to both.

QUALITY

Quality is a must for work related to medicines for the treatment of disease. The quality of intermediates and active ingredients have to meet the product and the regulatory authorities' requirements. The production standards have to meet the levels demanded. This is a must and is easily checked by customer and external audits. A supplier will not only accept but also ask to be audited because such an audit and its results assure that internal company perceptions and the external reality are in line with each other.

Quality changes during upscaling are very important to monitor. Often the first samples have a better purity than the material made later on during the upscaling process. Even when a chemical synthesis is investigated thoroughly on the laboratory scale, it does not automatically assure the absence of surprises during upscaling. Some effects might only be detected above a certain production volume and some by-products might be formed only on larger scale. This is an intrinsic problem that the industry has to deal with, and nothing special in the interaction between two companies.

At the start of development, no real specification can be given or set and the companies have to work on the basis of samples' quality and the general quality requirements of the authorities. Often the analytical methods are developed in parallel while the project moves on. Within the same company, it is easy to agree to a special procedure and the exchange of even preliminary information is easy. However, once an external partner becomes involved, it tends to become more complex and difficult; at the end of some steps, somebody will write a bill and ask for money. Within a company, in theory, it is the same, but a normal part of a budgeting process. The colleagues will be compensated, even if they did not achieve a milestone. This is in contrast to an external partner like a chemical company, somebody will write an invoice and somebody else will receive it and approve it for release. Therefore, more general and also legal aspects have to be considered, and one aspect is clearly measurable quality.

Disagreement over quality might lead to claims, and one part of an agreement will be analytical results. These results will be used for approval or rejection of material. As rejection may well have financial consequences, analytical methods are very often a point of discussion. Different organizations deal differently with this situation. Some share all analytical methods, samples, and data without any problem, while others are extremely restrictive with such information. Some companies request detailed and strong confidentiality agreements (CDAs) while others are more flexible. Depending on the wording of a CDA, such an agreement might be not acceptable to a supplier because it might bind the supplier even beyond the life of a project and restrict future business opportunities. Therefore, again depending on the customer's organization, the interactions are more or less easy. Sometimes, for business reasons, analytical methods have to be reinvented, which is time consuming and a waste of time and money. Other organizations see it more pragmatically and transfer methods to their suppliers even in an early stage of the project when a method is barely more than an idea of how the analytical methods might eventually emerge. Most chemical companies are not sellers of analytical equipment or methods, and therefore it is hard to see why for some organizations it is so essential to keep methods during a development phase in-house and to add costs to projects.

Besides product quality, there are other factors of quality. Keeping timelines is also a part of the overall quality. Time is money, especially in the pharmaceutical industry investing hundreds of millions in the development of a single new drug while running against the patent expiry date. Time counts twice. So, to keep chemical development off the critical path of the project is part of the project manager's duties. It will be true for the supplier as well and the ability to deliver not only in spec and in full but also on time is clearly an important factor for the overall performance. Also, at the supplier's end, the project will have a critical path and the supplier's project manager will have to manage the project in a way that it does not violate the pharma project's critical path. To have the right picture it is necessary to share all relevant information.

COMMERCIAL EXPECTATIONS

Service providers are not nonprofit organizations. They have shareholders and they have to deliver profit or else they will disappear. The same is true for the pharmaceutical industry. Even virtual pharma companies, in a phase of cash burn, have dreams of becoming profitable and to earn money by royalties or product sales after the phase of development. However, the margin expectations of chemical companies are lower than the margin pharmaceutical companies expect, and this is the commercial motivator for outsourcing activities. When the partners share this point of view, big hurdles can be cleared. Some years ago, there was the expectation from various pharma companies to get services free of charge and to squeeze the suppliers as hard as possible. The resulting shake-out of the industry that started then is still not over. The automotive industry did the same but the results are now apparent: The quality of some cars is now so bad that the reputation of their manufacturers has been damaged.

We have seen in recent years more and more companies entering the field of formerly high-margin businesses and, correspondingly, the financial figures of many companies eroded. At the same time, companies in China and India have emerged offering products at prices not achievable based on western production costs. This has speeded up the process of consolidation in the industry. Today, the first signals for consolidation are also visible in India and China, and the local Asian markets are battlefields with no mercy.

For the pharmaceutical industry, the opportunities are enormous and a lot of buyers grab for them. For the project managers, the situation has become more complex; having potential development partners in different parts of the world might be an advantage. However, the expectation to get Asian prices with western standards out of a western company will never materialize. Only when both parties agree to cooperate on a satisfactory commercial level will there be a partnership. This should be accepted by both sides.

CONCLUSION

External companies supporting the development of a new drug may contribute to the development at a high level. Working with different organizations brings new challenges to the project manager, but it also broadens the available knowledge for a given question. To develop an understanding of the different drivers and motivators for the companies is at least as important as understanding the hard technical facts. Once two companies have managed to develop a good understanding, in other words, once the key drivers of a project have developed an excellent working relationship, it is unbelievable how a project can be speeded up.

To keep innovation rates high, the help of external partners offers the best option for any given organization. The management of such a project is more complex than a purely internal project, but with the right setup and the right partner this complexity pays off and the projects can be developed quickly and be highly successful.

REFERENCES

1. http://www.geert-hofstede.com. Accessed in July 2005.
2. Hofstede G. Cultures and Organizations. New York: McGraw-Hill, 2004.
3. Hofstede G. Cultures and Organizations. London: Profile Books, 1994.
4. Hofstede G. Uncommon Sense About Organizations: Cases, Studies, and Field Observations. London: Sage Publications, 1994.
5. Hofstede G. Masculinity and Femininity. London: Sage Publications, 1998.

6

Clinical Trials—Can They Be Project Managed?

Les Rose

Pharmavision Consulting Ltd., West Harnham, Salisbury, U.K.

THE CLINICAL RESEARCH LANDSCAPE

Drug development involves the translation of cutting-edge science into commercial reality by providing concrete healthcare benefits to the community. Demanding as the science is, clinical trials have more problems with management than with science. Indeed, in later-phase trials, the majority of project team members spend far more time on management and administration than they do on science. Over 20 years of training clinical research staff in project management, I have found that most trainees worry vastly more about missing time, cost, and quality targets than they do about unexpected scientific findings. Yet, I sometimes hear experienced people claiming that clinical trials are too unpredictable for detailed project management. My objective is to show that this is not the case. Indeed, the inherent variability and risk of biological systems demand the best project management practices available.

How Has the Territory Shifted?

Compared with what I said here in 1996, many things remain the same. The clinical phases of drug development still present some of the most serious tests of management skills. Compared with other high-technology industries, we have this curious conundrum. As our drug candidate passes along the development pathway, it demands rapidly escalating resources, in terms of labor and cost, and at the same time, much of the influence on progress is passed to external parties—the clinical investigators.

The Impact of Regulation

In other ways, things are very different. Clinical trials are vastly more complex now, especially because of much increased regulation. Although there has been a major effort to standardize practices via initiatives such as the International Conference on Harmonisation (ICH), the effect has been to add more layers of regulation triggering the need for more project oversight and compliance checking. This has made project plans, if they are ever built, longer and with more convoluted logical networks.

The Impact of Technology

In 1996, hardly anyone used teleconferences. Electronic data capture (EDC) was hardly used and the Internet was in its infancy. We mostly communicated by telephone and letter, and we generally had to travel to get decent information on progress. It is hard to quantify the effects of business technology on the project management of clinical trials. Any improvement we may have obtained from technology could well have been offset by the increased complexity of projects. We will look at both of these competing aspects later; suffice it to say at this stage that there is precious little to convince me that technology has generally improved time to market. There is quite a good argument that it might have had the opposite effect. If this is the case, it is a tragedy because business technology has always offered the potential of transforming the drug development process. This is to a large extent because clinical trials are extremely bureaucratic. Clinical research associates (CRAs) still spend a majority of their time doing essentially clerical work such as collecting and checking documents, checking data, and filing papers.

So What Is the State of the Art?

Drug Development Performance Indicators

Before considering how well project management is doing in this field, it is worth looking at how well drug development overall is doing. One of the most reputable sources of industry data is CMR International, which stated in 2007:

> "There is a continuing decline in productivity in the industry. In the last ten years, despite an approximate 70% increase in R&D expenditure, the output of new molecular entities (NMEs) has fallen by over 30% and only 15–20% of revenues are derived from products introduced in the past five years." (1)

For a cohort of companies accounting for 84% of the total global R&D expenditure, mean total development time was just under 11 years in 1998 and over 12 years in 2006. Clinical development accounts for half of this (Fig. 1) and the trend over time is clearly upwards (Fig. 2). This is despite the *improvements*

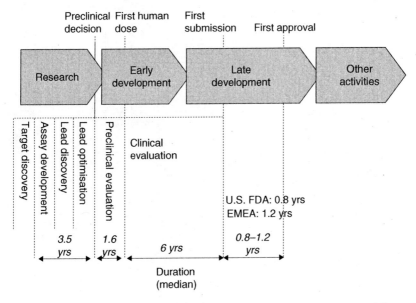

Figure 1 Overall drug development cycle time in 2006. *Source*: Courtesy of Centre for Medicines Research International, Epsom, UK. R&D e-Factbook, 2007. *Abbreviations*: FDA, Food and Drug Administration; EMEA, European Medicines Evaluation Agency.

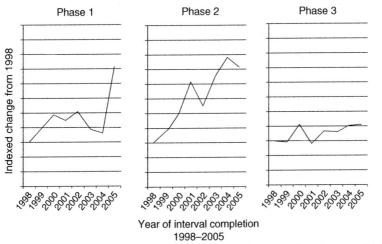

Data show the indexed change from 1998 in duration for four intervals for each year. Intervals were completed in the year shown, where the start and end milestone dates for the interval were available.

Figure 2 There are convincing indications that cycle times are likely to continue to increase. *Source*: Courtesy of Centre for Medicines Research International, Epsom, UK. R&D e-Factbook, 2007.

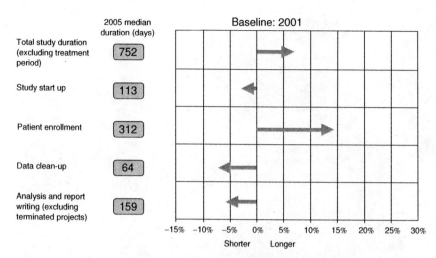

The percentage change data presented in this graph are baseed on data provided for all years by a consistant cohort of 23 companies (12 Major, 4 Mid, and 7 Other companies). Data shows percentage change for median duration from 2001 to 2005 for Phase 2 (excluding Phase 1 in patients) and 3 clinical studies that completed the named interval in that year. During data are shown for studies where data for all milestone dates for the interval are available. For the "Analysis and report writing" interval studies where the project was terminated prior to completion of the final integrated report are excluded.

Figure 3   Changes in clinical trial key stages, 2001–2005. *Source*: Courtesy of Centre for Medicines Research International, Epsom, UK. R&D e-Factbook, 2007.

in regulatory approval times for all three ICH regions over the same period. But CMR has another interesting message:

> "Major companies have shorter development cycle times than do smaller companies, and the gap is widening. The expanding range of cycle times suggests that some companies have found ways to shorten the development time."

So what have some companies discovered that others have not? Let us not get too excited. There have been markedly increased cycle times all round for phases 1 and 2 suggesting that more effort is being invested in early decision making while, as we have seen, overall time to market continues to rise.

The Contribution from Clinical Trials

Of all the R&D stages, clinical trials absorb, by far, the largest slice of resources—34% of the total. The median duration of a single trial is over two years. Of the generally accepted milestones within phase 2 and 3 trials, between 2001 and 2005, only data cleanup and analysis and report writing improved significantly—by only seven and six percent respectively (Fig. 3). Patient enrolment time increased by 14% contributing the largest part of an overall increase in trial duration of 17%. These figures make it clear therefore that clinical trials should be a major target for improvement. It appears that sponsors are having a positive effect on the activities that are within their control, which is mitigating, to some extent, the continuing deterioration in other activities. Let us at this point reflect that for a phase 3 trial with a typical total duration of two years, 10% lateness represents in the region of US $50 to 100 million of lost sales, because of delay to market. Add all that up for the whole clinical trial program and we are looking at potentially crippling losses.

Are Clinical Research Projects Really Different?

Many specialists are convinced that they have unique problems not seen in other fields. Clinical trials do have particular difficulties. Scientific risk is commonly cited as a cardinal feature of drug development, in general, and clinical trials, in particular. However, people from the petrochemical industry do not find that unusual. Oil exploration carries huge geological risks with only a small proportion of drilled wells becoming productive. Civil engineering tells a similar story, as those building bridges and tunnels will confirm. Therefore, I do not think that excessive risk marks out clinical trials as especially difficult projects.

Is heavy regulation the problem? I have already linked this with an increased complexity, but again, other industries are very tightly regulated. Construction is beset with planning and building regulations as well as onerous health and safety regulations. Heavy industry of all types is now having to comply with much increased environmental and consumer regulation. We in clinical research have a particular kind of regulation but other industries have their own and, in that, we are not alone.

But, what other high-technology products are developed by effectively farming out the work to a vast international network of essentially amateur researchers? It was this to which I alluded earlier—the increasing delegation of the work to external team members while at the same time escalating the scope and cost (Fig. 4). An outside observer would quite rightly think of this as a recipe for disaster and it is probably one of the key features of clinical research. I do not know of another industry that does this on such a scale; it forms a large part of the major challenge facing the clinical project manager.

As if this were not worrying enough, there is another difference, which I think is of the industry's own making. It is a cultural and organizational issue, which I want to analyze in more detail later, but to which I should alert you now. Compared with other industries, project managers in drug development are much less empowered. Line management in many companies still dominates. This can readily be seen by looking at job advertisements. Curiously, project managers in engineering may be less well-qualified scientifically but have more financial responsibility and more authority. There are other cultural differences that lead to damaging habits; these will emerge in later pages.

The purpose of this brief analysis is not to denigrate a successful industry; rather, in the spirit of continuous improvement, we should look at how best practice can be approached.

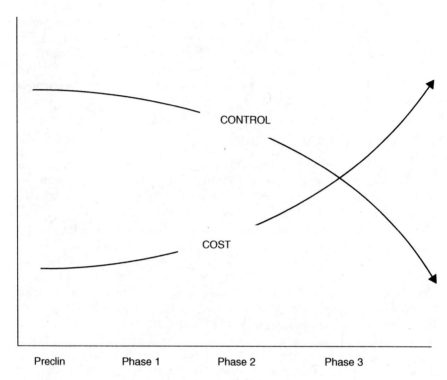

Preclin   Phase 1   Phase 2   Phase 3

Figure 4   Schematic representation of the clinical trial cost-control paradox.

PROJECT MANAGEMENT BEST PRACTICE IN A CLINICAL RESEARCH CONTEXT

Is the Current Practice Realistic?

There is a widespread management technique that imposes impossible goals, with no expectation that they will be achieved. What the proponents of this method do expect is that another goal, secret and less demanding, will be achieved; the logic is that people will respond to unreasonable pressure by working harder than they would do if the target were realistic. You will not find this idea in any serious book about management, for the simple reason that it does not work; people are demoralized by a continual sense of failure and do not respect unattainable objectives. Yet, I have worked for companies that practiced this and I have many consultancy clients who are its victims.

This point is made to emphasize that the fundamentals of good project management are dealing openly with people on a realistic basis. In clinical trials, there are special reasons for adhering to these principles. Increasing complexity has multiplied the number of specialisms within the project team, thus increasing the range of negotiations that have to be carried out during the planning process, and later when the study or program of studies is under way.

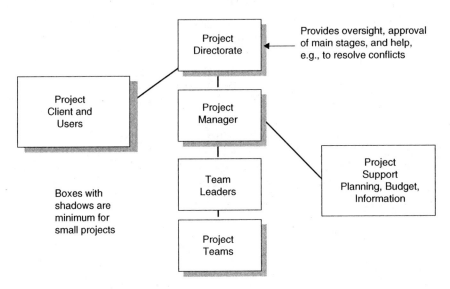

Figure 5 Typical project organization. *Source*: Courtesy of Centre for Medicines Research International, Epsom, UK. R&D e-Factbook, 2007.

The Multidisciplinary Team

The traditional core roles of pharmaceutical physician and CRA have proliferated substantially in recent years. Fifteen years ago, a typical team might have comprised these two along with internal support and administration staff, all interacting with the study-site personnel, usually starting with the clinician who has the overall authority for the site. Other study-site personnel included research nurses, study-site coordinators, technicians, junior medical staff, and administrative staff (e.g., medical secretaries). Other disciplines within or connected to the site's institution included pharmacists, laboratory staff, and ethics committees. This was complex enough at the time. Now we have institutional research and development committees and in many countries two levels of ethics committees, specialist committees such as those for gene therapy and radioactive substances, and a host of other specialists and groups according to the type of trial. Exacerbating the complexity of negotiations is the minimal control that the project manager has over some external areas such as patient recruitment or ethics committee approval.

Customers (or Clients), Sponsors, and Stakeholders

Figure 5 shows a simplified organization chart for a project based on the PRINCE2 methodology (2). Many companies are now operating a customer-orientated culture that helps to clarify for whom any work is being done. A project starts with the customer or client—who issues an initial requirement—and it is vital to be clear as to who this is. For a registration package of studies, the client could be the regulatory department, but might it not also be the marketing department, which will have to use the data? Other potential clients are the regulatory authorities who issue specifications as to how the data should be submitted, the investigators who will be using the drug, and let us not forget the patients! Thus, the more we look, the more complex the situation appears—with great potential for a communication breakdown and project failure.

Much of this risk can be avoided by carrying out the right analysis at the outset. We live in an age pervaded by jargon and the word stakeholder is common currency. In the present context, it means anyone who has something to gain out of the project. I could challenge the reader to identify anyone involved who has nothing to gain! The stakeholder analysis can be especially valuable for clinical trials. Identifying stakeholder motivation can make the difference between success and failure. A good example is the perennial problem of patient recruitment in the hands, as we know, of external investigators. When we recruit investigators, do we know what their motivation is? It may not be what we thought and we are not going to find out without asking.

With regard to clients, contract research organizations (CROs) have some advantages in that they are usually clear as to who their client is. This is not because it is always obvious from the start but because they have to be clear or any negotiation is useless. The problems really occur when the apparent client is later found to lack the authority for key decisions, so a careful review of plans and especially decision points is needed and the correct responsibility needs to be assigned to each stage. The point here is the difference between the client as a company and the key individuals and functional areas within it.

Now, in many pharmaceutical companies (and companies serving them), there may well be some overlap in function between what I describe as the client and what is now identified as the project sponsor. A widely accepted definition of this role is: An active senior management role responsible for identifying the business need, problem, or opportunity. The sponsor ensures that the project remains a viable proposition and that benefits are realized resolving any issues that are outside the control of the project manager (3).

It is important to distinguish between the two meanings of the word "sponsor." One is the drug regulatory meaning and the other is the project meaning. A major problem for many organizations is that this role was never defined. It is particularly relevant today in that a large proportion of clinical development is contracted out to CROs. While the latter may clearly identify their client's sponsorship role, they need to consider that they also have (or should have) their own internal sponsor. This is because the two roles have different objectives. For example, the client wishes to minimize costs whereas the CRO wishes to maximize them. There is nothing underhand about this; it is just normal business. In fact, many CROs will agree that a significant proportion of revenue is made from contract modifications, which will attract a great deal of negotiation effort by both client and CRO sponsors.

Current Standards of Project Planning

The complexity of relationships within and close to the project team, which we have examined here, implies that the project plans are going to be complex. So far, no consensus seems to have emerged. One feature, however, is very clear. Standards of planning are generally far lower in clinical trials than they are in other industries. It could well be that the great complexity discourages detailed planning—it is just too much hard work. Clinical project managers have often told me that. One cause of this seems to be very short lead times. It is common for a pivotal study to be given approval to start planning with less than three months before first patient entry. For CROs, this can be much worse with sponsors delaying approval to start to such an extent that a new project manager may find himself/herself already working on deliverables when planning has hardly started. Other industries usually devote far more time to project definition and planning.

But I am probably describing one end of the capability spectrum. There is, in fact, a wide variation between companies regarding their development cycle times, as shown in Figure 6. Some are getting it right, some are getting it wrong. The implication is that some are better at planning than others.

So, how can we plan realistically? How can we rely on the information we obtain from all these people and build it into an effective plan? Let us start with the client, who issues the requirement for the clinical trial(s) and uses the results. If requirements were always clear to everyone, planning would be far easier than it often is; but, to a great extent, the time-honored methodology for protocol development does not always give good results. Figure 7 shows the typical stages that a proposal goes through before culminating in an approved protocol. Naturally, detail level increases as the study proposal develops, with very little detail in the top-level development plan. At this level, only outline estimates of time and cost are possible but at least one target must be clearly defined. This is what we expect the drug to do, embodied in the target product profile (4). It is important to emphasize that although this may be quite extensively defined at the outset it will most likely have to change as more is discovered about the drug. This concept is not exclusively the province of clinical trials but since we are testing the drug in humans for the first time, we are going to be finding out the most relevant information for its eventual marketing. Thus the top-level plan and the clinical development plan that emanates from it will map out trials designed to contribute to the target product profile. As the latter changes, the types of studies we actually do may well change. This is just one of the many feedback loops involved in protocol development, and which to my mind are insufficiently considered.

It is rare for a protocol to have no amendments and common for many drafts to be written. What, for example, happens if the initial requirement is incomplete? Can we assume safely that the client has (i) thought of everything he/she needs and (ii) effectively communicated these needs in the requirement? Yet, the conventional process makes just this assumption, with the result that gaps can remain unfilled or, perhaps even worse, be filled erroneously by people further down the chain.

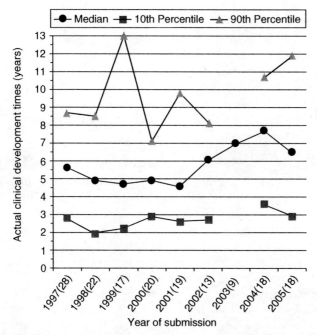

Actual clinical development time is calculated for lead projects as the time between "First human dose" and "First submission". Data represent all lead projects that reached "First submission" between 1997–2005, where the start and end milestone dates for the interval are available. (n) = number of projects analysed in each year. Data for the 10th percentile and 90th percentile are shown where n ≥ 10.

Figure 6 Clinical development times have increased but there is considerable variability between companies. *Source*: Courtesy of Centre for Medicines Research International, Epsom, UK. R&D e-Factbook, 2007.

A second common problem with protocols is the lack of focus on functional objectives. For example, a clear objective would be "to enable a decision on which patient population to target in the marketing campaign". A less clear objective would be "to evaluate the safety and efficacy of . . ." The first offers a clear benefit from a successful trial, the second does not—if the drug turns out to be safe and effective (and we need criteria here), what are we going to do with the knowledge? This exemplifies the need for clear thinking and structured communication, usually with a wide range of people directly or indirectly involved in the trial.

Study Designs and Methods

The reasons for so much protocol change appear to cover the full range, from reliance on well-established designs without allowing newer, more creative ideas to be considered, to failing to test new methods for the current application. For example, in an angina study, treadmill exercise testing was used as the primary efficacy criterion. This is, of course, an extremely well-validated methodology but in this

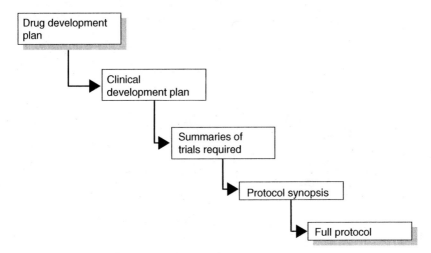

Figure 7   Main stages in protocol development.

case the patients were elderly, so the exercise protocol was substantially modified to reduce the physical demand. The problem was that with such a mild exercise protocol, less than half the patients recruited showed sufficient electrocardiogram changes to qualify for randomization. A quick pilot study would have alerted the sponsors before committing to major cost.

These problems, of which the foregoing is only a very small selection, exemplify how important the definition stage is for clinical trials as projects. As I write, I am assisting a sponsor with an international phase 3 program in which the final deliverable has not yet been fully defined. Several trials are under way but it is impossible to fix a target date for final delivery because we do not know the scope of one of the key deliverables. Yes, we do know when we *must* complete but we do not know how realistic that date is. We could find ourselves overspending unnecessarily if the scope turns out to be less than what we thought. There seems often to be insufficient attention paid to defining business outcomes, which is surprising in view of the technical field we are in. Clinical research specialists are usually not admitted to discussions about the commercial value of the studies they are managing, which is odd in view of how close to market this development stage is.

Clinical Trial Planning in Context

Planning Structures and Templates—Programs and Subprojects

So far, I have not defined what I mean by a "project" in the clinical trials context. The answer is that it is whatever you, the reader, want it to mean. Figure 8 shows a hierarchy of different levels of project management. At the top is the whole company portfolio, with each bar in the Gantt chart representing one compound

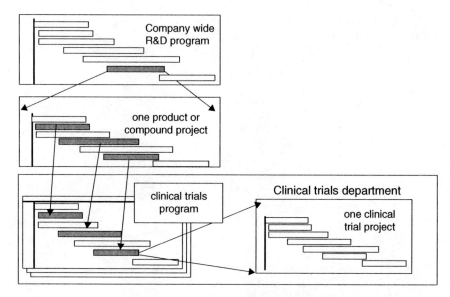

Figure 8 Levels of project planning in drug development. *Source*: Courtesy of Centre for Medicines Research International, Epsom, UK. R&D e-Factbook, 2007.

project. Below that is the drug development project for a compound, containing several subprojects, some of which will be clinical trials. These can be aggregated into the clinical development program or project shown below that. Finally, each clinical trial itself will be managed as its own project. It is important to remember that the same skills are used, irrespective of the level we are looking at. Now my experience is that many companies today are good at planning their portfolios, quite good at planning their compound projects, but not good at planning individual clinical trials. The rigor and detail of planning declines as one goes down the levels. But, consider this: The purpose of the plan is to create a tool for control. The clinical trials themselves are the crucial level—this is where the work is done and data are captured. If we do not plan in detail at this level, how can we have control at the top level?

The Role of Senior Management

Of course, senior management will be looking at the top-level plan much more closely than they do at the individual trial level. But, the costs and risks of failure in the clinical phases are so large that they should be occupying much of top management's attention. Yet, in many companies, requirements, objectives, budgets, and deadlines are imposed without any negotiation. On top of this, major changes are commonly dictated by management, usually by changing priorities. How can the clinical project manager fulfill top management's aspirations within an increasingly constrained environment? I alluded earlier to certain cultural features of pharmaceutical companies that delineate them from other high-technology industries and this line-management-dominated structure is a cardinal one.

Predicting the (Apparently) Unpredictable—Managing Risk

All research and development must involve some risk. Apart from scientific and technical risks, operational risks will include rejection of submissions for approvals (ethics, regulatory, and, now in the United Kingdom, institutional research and development committees), study sites that do not perform and drop out, and protocols with flaws that compromise study conduct. It is not necessary to itemize here a full list of potential risks—the reader will be well aware of them. My purpose here is to highlight the need for some sort of systematic approach to managing risk, which I find is all too rare. Again, there may be a cultural background to this. Let me give you two anecdotes by way of illustration. The first concerns a sponsor who invited tenders from CROs to run a multicenter trial. One CRO tried to follow the best practice and included a detailed risk-management plan. This so terrified the sponsor that they rejected the proposal. They really did not want to contemplate the idea that anything could go wrong. The other concerns a sponsor who had appointed a CRO to run a phase 1 study. At the first meeting, the sponsor asked about risk management. The CRO did not understand. So, the sponsor simply asked, "What can go wrong with this study?" The answer came quickly: "Why, nothing will go wrong." Of course, something did go wrong and the CRO learned a valuable lesson. I think it is very important that we put in place some sort of methodology for dealing with risk. Whatever is used, it will almost certainly be better than doing no risk assessment at all, which is more often the case.

I just want to leave this topic with one key point. Risk management is what we do before starting the project. It is a planning activity but is often misunderstood. Yes, new problems arise during the project but I prefer to call these issues. They are actually things that we should have predicted and confusing the two mitigates against good project control. However, valuable as proactive risk management is, it cannot be perfect. Normal practice is to brainstorm all possible risks and only to plan action for the most likely and the most damaging. This is the usual probability times the impact calculation. Done properly, this will deal with most risks but, during the project, we will get problems from risks we originally thought unlikely and from others that we missed. That is life.

Risk Distribution in Clinical Phases

Delivering the results on time and to the required standard may have a lower risk in phase 1 than in later phases, mainly because subjects are healthy and not potentially complicated patients, and thus recruitment can be predicted with some confidence. However, first administration to humans is something of a leap into the unknown and safety problems are always to be considered. What is possibly less obvious is the risk to later phases and to the whole drug project resulting from early-phase design errors. Recently, this has been graphically illustrated by the unprecedented serious adverse events experienced in one first-in-human study in the United Kingdom. Much has been written about this, which I do not intend to repeat, but I am convinced that there are management as well as scientific issues arising. I have already highlighted the need for rigorous project definition; one lesson learned from this tragic episode (in which six healthy volunteers suffered, to various extents, serious injury and disability) was that there was insufficient consideration of all the alternative approaches that might have been used (5). There is a solution to this, which we will look at later.

As we enter phase 2, we need to remember that there is a much greater risk than ever that the drug will not progress beyond this point. This is where top management must, well in advance, decide on the criteria for success. However, quite commonly, the outcome of a phase 2a proof-of-concept trial falls short of expectation; yet, no clear decision is made. Yes, it is hard to give up on a compound that we have nurtured through the preclinical stage and phase 1, but if it simply does not perform in the clinic, it is only going to cause more problems later on and, of course, cause wastage of money. Again, planning is the key and, in this case, I like the question "What does success look like?" This is the question that has to be asked at clinical development plan stage and not forgotten as we get embroiled in the detail of individual studies.

Once phase 3 is imminent, there is perhaps a degree of confidence emerging as much more is known about the drug. The requirement for phase 3 may therefore be seen as accumulating data to enable a product license application. In fact, the great expansion of activity dictated by phase 3 studies introduces even more complexity and a new set of risks. The application of the drug to a more realistic clinical setting means that we will not necessarily be studying "clean" patients— they will often have other diseases on top of that under study and will only be under observation for a small proportion of the time. Attention to protocol design is thus at least as critical as in phases 1 and 2.

We should not forget phase 4 studies, which have actually expanded substantially in recent years. In general, they are exposed to similar risks as phase 3 and, indeed, are more similar now in that they are subject to uniform regulation under ICH, GCP, and EU legislation.

Key Tasks at Project Start

The most common reason for tasks and projects finishing late is that they started late. Before patients can be screened for entry, a well-established set of startup tasks must be completed and, of these, some are relatively easy to plan while others are less predictable. Those relying on internal agreements (e.g., drug supplies, protocol sign-off) can be expedited by instilling the right culture of negotiation between departments and individuals. But what of the external elements, particularly regulatory and ethics approvals? I am going to consider all types of approvals together for the moment as, although they are technically different, they can benefit from similar approaches. I am also going to focus on later-stage trials, particularly international ones, because they exemplify many of the difficulties we can face. We are all familiar, as has been mentioned earlier, with attempts to standardize regulation. Within the EU, North America, and Japan, we all follow the ICH guidelines and, within the EU, we now have the Clinical Trials Directive and the Good Clinical Practice Directive, both enacted into the national law within most member states at the time of writing. We might expect these overarching regulations to standardize much of what goes on but, in practice, there remains a huge geographical variation. In some EU countries, ethics committee submissions must be made after regulatory submissions while, in some, they must be done together and there are various permutations involving different rules on time scales. These rules seem to change frequently. This can make planning a nightmare unless an effort is put into keeping planning information totally up to date. I have recently had the experience of using approved planning templates for an EU study within a very large organization only to be told by the CRA in one country that the template is wrong because the rules have changed. The message here is that investment in an accurate and up-to-date planning information is vital. It has a major bearing on what countries you might consider for your international program.

Quantity, Quality, Timeliness

Any discussion of clinical research planning and conduct sooner or later gravitates to the question of patient recruitment. We have already seen that patient recruitment time has increased substantially over recent years (Fig. 3). How realistically one can plan for recruitment depends very much on the type of study. For a stable chronic disease, such as essential hypertension, large volumes of data should be available to enable good estimates of the number of patients expected. This will come from medical practitioners' records but it is vital that any estimating database is modified for the current study. What the investigator observes is not that all the patients of hypertension disappear—there are just as many as ever—but that he had not applied the selection criteria when estimating recruitment. Most experienced managers have learned to apply big discounts to investigators' estimates of patient availability. Sophisticated computer modeling now enables a better prediction of recruitment and provides better monitoring during the recruitment, and specialist recruitment companies have sprung into being, yet still across the industry it is getting worse not better.

For acute diseases, there is a higher risk of recruitment estimates being inaccurate as one is relying on new cases arising with a predictable frequency. For instance, some conditions are strongly seasonal and some seasons will be better (or worse) than others; so, it is vital to retrieve data far enough back in time to avoid being misled by an unusually high-prevalence season. Even if we are reassured by this, we should still ask the all-important project manager's question "What happens if . . .?" and, in this case, "What happens if the next season is unusually benign?"

Protocol Compliance

We have considered earlier, the challenge of achieving a protocol that will not need to be amended. Even if we meet this challenge, the next one is to ensure compliance. If the protocol is difficult to follow and even if we have no problems in finding patients (a rare scenario), there is still the great danger of many of these patients being invalidated by protocol violations because the drug is now being used in the real world of clinical medicine. If it is critical that clinic assessments are carried out at particular times of day (e.g., to coincide with trough drug levels or to plot the time course of postdose response), how confident can we be that this will be observed? Can we measure the impact on the study of exceptions to the rule? Can we estimate how many valid patients we might lose? Please remember that in this section I am not providing solutions, just painting a picture of the clinical research landscape. These are factors that need to be considered when planning.

The Data Cleaning Cycle

We may not only lose data because of protocol violations. Quality of work varies widely between centers, so what contingency should we include to allow for query resolution and consequent delays to database lock? With most companies maintaining records of investigator performance, this is critical information to include. If queries are being tracked electronically, it is relatively simple to generate statistics on data query incidence and turn-round. However, these are traditionally used mainly to feed back performance data to centers during the study rather than for planning new projects. Detailed information on the study-center quality performance is a powerful planning tool. I can remember excluding some high-recruiting centers from new studies because the protocol compliance and data quality were so poor that many patients recruited were invalid. Interestingly, there is no evidence that the so-called centers of excellence, the high-profile teaching hospital units, are any better in this regard and their quality performance is usually inferior to a well-trained general practice center.

Clinical Trial Risk Management—A Summary

Clearly, any detailed examination of clinical trial risks could fill a whole chapter and here we have discussed just some of those that routinely catch my attention. This section has no doubt raised more questions than answers and this, indeed, is the essence of the message; unless the project manager asks the questions based on "What happens if . . .?," the most elegant of plans will be vulnerable to sudden and unexpected change or will be destroyed altogether. Perhaps this is why 90% of project management software purchasers just use it to do initial planning and never update their plans—it would be too disappointing if they did!

Getting More from Less—Multiple Projects, Priorities, Workload, and Progress Control

All the complexity described so far would apply even if each person were involved with only one clinical trial. The reality is that most people are doing all this for several trials, multiplying the problems and introducing new ones. This is substantially different from where project management grew up, in construction and engineering. The generally accepted view is of a manager responsible for one project, although this may be anything from the local apartment block to the

Channel Tunnel. Thus, clinical research should be in the forefront of developing new project management approaches in a high-risk industry.

The Need for Policies on Prioritization

To get some sense out of conflicting multiple clinical trials, some form of prioritization is necessary and it helps to reduce this to as simple a level as possible. One company was accustomed to assigning individual priority levels to all its clinical trials so that there might be as many as 40 levels. The problem was that no one could remember the actual priority of each study, so levels were not adhered to and were open to change without notice by senior management. Because so many other factors can influence the sequencing of trials, holding some up and releasing others, it is perfectly possible to manage them with as few as three priority levels (although some of the software systems confusingly allow many levels). Project managers and team members regularly tell me that priorities are constantly changing, causing discontinuities triggered by switching work from project to project. CROs are particularly vulnerable to this. They usually have a large portfolio of totally unrelated projects, commissioned by different clients. Each client thinks that its project is top priority and will bring pressure to bear for immediate action if things appear to be running late. A frequent solution is to switch more resource to the project that is in trouble. Not only does this compromise other projects (they start to run late because of reduced resource) but the very act of switching ties up the resource itself. This is because work has to be handed over and new staff brought up to a suitable level of competence. I am convinced that constant switching of staff is one of the most damaging activities in clinical trials, especially in CROs.

Priority or Urgency?

Although much of the industry's focus regarding risk is on drug safety crises, the great interest in the concept shows how much we tend to enjoy an emergency— team spirit is always high and there is a great sense of achievement at the end. Often the problem is not a genuinely unforeseeable one arising externally but simply a conflict of priorities. For example, if one clinical trial is running late and another is scheduled to start immediately as soon as the staff is available from completing the first, the second is delayed because of the need to finish the first. This then feeds through the whole program until all the projects are late and thus managed as crises. A better technique is to recognize the high priority of trial 1 at the outset and do everything possible to complete it on time, even if this means extra staff or some other expense. This then breaks the vicious circle of crisis feeding crisis. An additional benefit is that if projects are scheduled sequentially rather than in parallel the total investment is less and profitability is higher. This works in the following way. If two projects are conducted at once, there can be no return on investment until they are both completed. If however one project is held up and twice the effort is put into the other, cash flow starts earlier, maximum investment is less (because the first helps to pay for the second), yet the second project is no later in completing (Fig. 9). To put this into a clinical trial perspective, should

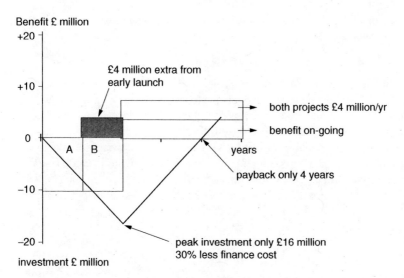

Figure 9 Cash benefit of doing projects in series, not in parallel. *Source*: Courtesy of Centre for Medicines Research International, Epsom, UK. R&D e-Factbook, 2007.

you try to run two phase 3 anti-infective programs at the same time? You might do better to put all your skilled people and budget on one of them, run twice as many study centers, and finish it earlier. An early launch will win you more patent protection and help you get in front of more of your competitors. The second program will be no later than if you had run them at the same time. Some readers may think this to be a difficult tool to use, when payback from a project may take a long time to appear in premarketing development, but what about phase 4? If we are running a study to provide more confidence to the prescribers of the drug in the clinic, it is entirely feasible to get those results published quickly, especially in this age of the Web-based publication. In fact, it is what is expected of drug companies today.

Progress Information—Can We Believe It?

If you have read this far, you will see that project management software can be far more than just a planning tool. You can be updating your plans to give you ongoing control of your clinical trials. Indeed, software does not manage projects, only people do. To do this, reliable information on the study progress is needed, and the word "reliable" is vital. There continues to be, to my mind, a disproportionate amount of attention paid to patient recruitment, almost as if it were the only deliverable that matters. It is often not properly defined. For example, is there physical evidence of the clean case report forms in-house? Unproven information may still be useful for giving early warning of problems, but should not be relied upon for reporting progress to senior management.

For a number of reasons, normal practice now is to track all the many tasks and elements in a trial using a proliferating number of computer spreadsheets. This practice stems from the ease with which spreadsheets can be used and the difficulty of managing detailed tracking information in most project management software. The danger is that spreadsheets proliferate uncontrollably as one team member after another discovers something else that has not been tracked so far. I know of team members who are automatically e-mailed various sheets at regular intervals, without knowing why. The trap into which many managers fall is that of information overload and this extends outside the project team too.

People in Projects

Senior Management Revisited

Reports to management tend to consume huge amounts of effort. I know of one country affiliate that was required to send a clinical research report to its overseas head office and this report ran to at least 80 pages every month. Much of the information was repeated from previous months and all the multitude of details could not be read by all the recipients—they would never have the time. The key to effective reporting lies with the project manager, who must get agreement on what information is necessary and when.

The Tyranny of the Teleconference

Believe it or not, there was a time when clinical trials could be effectively managed without today's obligatory (and multiple) weekly teleconferences. For some reason, it is now considered that these can solve all sorts of problems as if by magic. This is not a joke. On one occasion, I found myself pitched into the first weekly gathering over the ether, with no briefing, no training, and yet somehow expected to make decisions. The problem with these actually valuable business tools is that they are much too easy to abuse. What is the point of heading an agenda thus? "Meeting Purpose: Weekly Global Teleconference".

This is from a real clinical program. No, this is not the purpose, it is the label. Unless objectives are properly defined, meaningful decisions are unlikely. What actually happens is that these events are filled up with people from around the world telling everyone else what they have been doing, when in reality only a minority need to know and the information could have been transmitted before the event. Because people commonly have teleconferences stacked up throughout the day, if anyone does start to discuss a problem needing resolution there is rarely enough time to do so before the next alarm goes off on everyone's computer.

Multidisciplinary Team-Working

We have already considered the multidisciplinary nature of modern drug development. So diverse are the skills required that the understanding between the skill holders may be incomplete. Therefore, the project manager needs to be a generalist with appreciation (but not necessarily in-depth understanding) of a wide range of technical issues. This has benefits over time as well as horizontally. Transfer of data from one development stage to the next is less successful if the authority is transferred abruptly at the same time—continuity is essential. One approach, which has been used in passing manufacturing methods from phase 1 onwards, is to involve the later phase specialists as observers and advisers in the early phase teams, and vice versa. However, the key lies in lines of authority—to whom should the project managers report? I believe that they should report to the top management. If they report to anyone else, how can their authority be seen to be real?

Managing Contractors

Projects in engineering and construction are usually set up as extensive networks of contractors and subcontractors. Over the last 20 years, this model has become almost the norm for clinical trials. Clinical CROs are thus continuing to expand while a range of specialist vendors has come onto the stage. A few examples are central laboratories, EDC, interactive voice response systems (IVRS), and drug packaging and deployment. At the planning stage, decisions have to be made as to how this network is to be managed. To a large extent, it depends on the client's capabilities. Let us consider two options at either end of a continuum. One option is to find a full service CRO and delegate the whole lot to them. This will require very careful checking of all the services offered. Is their IVRS state of the art? Is their central laboratory fully accredited? The other option I have in mind is to engage all the vendors separately. This way, the client takes on all the work of managing the individual vendors' deliverables, and the interfaces between them. So, a small client company with few qualified staff would be unwise to choose the second option. However, here we encounter a dilemma. This option may be cheaper because we are not getting the CRO to do all this management. But, the small company may not be able to justify to the senior management the extra cost of the full service CRO. This is not the part of the chapter where I was intending to provide answers to dilemmas such as this but, to be honest, there is no easy answer. I am just highlighting the problem and showing that one needs to be clear on the options before committing to one of them. Too often, a modus operandi just develops from short-term expediency instead of from a clear strategy. I make no apology for drawing yet another comparison with nonpharmaceutical projects. These usually have extensive purchasing plans and clear operating procedures for dealing with contractors. The result is that such projects meet more of their targets and have fewer disputes over contracts.

The landscapes I have painted here are drawn from real life. They are not simply invented to dramatize points of argument. Modern clinical research is, on the whole, not badly conducted and, indeed, I never cease to be impressed with the dedication, professionalism, and sheer hard work of these thousands of people who are striving to obtain scientific evidence that we can believe. But we could do so much better.

THIS NEW WORLD OF CLINICAL RESEARCH

In 1996, this section talked about all the new and exciting things we could do to improve clinical research project management. This time, it has two themes: how much of what we wanted then has appeared and how much we can still do. I would like to kick off with the idea that was at the very end of the first edition of the chapter.

Slipping Through the Net

There can be no doubt that the Internet and specifically the World Wide Web, has had a pervasive and huge global impact. That it had the potential to revolutionize clinical trials was very obvious and a good deal of that expectation has been realized. In a document-dominated operating environment, the ability to compress many cycle times dramatically should be of massive value. We can now get protocol versions back and forth, several times a day, probably knocking weeks off study startup time. Or does it? Look again at Figure 1 and consider how much faster these activities really are. They are only about 3% faster than they were five years ago. On the other hand, with all the additional approval hurdles to overcome, let us thank the Web for coming to our rescue—things could have been far worse.

All organizations, independent of size, now work on a fully networked basis, although for many this remains quite haphazard. I still do not see the value of e-mailing documents as attachments to scores of people instead of keeping them centralized. This would not only economize on traffic but would also make version control more secure. However, I am much more surprised to find that a majority of trials are still carried out using paper case report forms. The technology for secure Web-based EDC has existed for a decade, confirming the innate conservatism of our industry. Moreover, the enormous potential of the Web, and particularly EDC, to enable real time project progress control remains seriously underexploited. This will only really happen when truly integrated information environments appear but, even in large and wealthy organizations (and perhaps especially in them), computer applications remain highly fragmented. Figure 10 gives examples, yet

- Trial management system
- Document management system
- Training system
- Investigator grants system
- Budget tracking
- Estimating database (time and cost)
- Time sheets
- Project management

Figure 10 Examples of unconnected software for clinical trials.

again drawn from a real company, of disparate systems with no interfaces between them other than manual updating of data by a hapless human—usually the project manager. It is not at all unusual for the same information to be entered into three different applications. For example, study-site address details might go into the trial management system, budget tracking, and investigator grants management. Study milestones will be set in both trial management and project management generating great effort in keeping them in agreement, as they change during the study's life cycle.

But I should suggest some solutions, as I promised. Software is moving much more towards open systems and it is easier now to set up data links between systems. People are beginning to take advantage of this, one good example being the dynamic updating of the patient recruitment tasks in the project system from spreadsheets of individually tracked patients. The immediate future lies not in building massive systems that do everything we can think of (but do not do the things other people thought of) but of interfacing what we have. That way, we could recover the control we lose when we delegate it to the external team members, who do not even see themselves as in a team at all.

The Cultural Dimension

The Web has already caused major cultural changes. In many ways, it has brought people closer together. We now mostly converse on first name terms, in a less formal manner, because that is the norm via e-mail. I genuinely find that there is a culture of mutual support and help across the Internet. This should make the project manager's job easier if people are that much more willing to help each other. But how many project managers agree with me?

Who Is the New Clinical Project Manager?

Despite these welcome trends, which I already identified in 1996 as moving towards a "flatter" management structure, today I still find that departmental heads generally have more status and benefits than project managers. My alternative view has not caught on; that clinical projects are so demanding that successfully completing them on time may be more difficult than running a department. This again contrasts starkly with other industries, which empower their project managers far more. But who are these project managers? By that I mean, do they really manage clinical trials as projects or are they really trial or study managers? I will try to explain what I mean by defining what a project manager really does.

Project Manager Functions

Potentially, there is no one better than a scientist for the project manager's role, because of his/her analytical approach to planning (and problems). This is more a valuable by-product of being a scientist than the main reason for the qualification, which is to have enough knowledge to assess that what one is being told is true— vital at the planning stages. However, it is hardly practical to engage a technical specialist to manage every new project; indeed, it is not necessary. In fact, there is a valid case that the project manager should be a generalist not a specialist. The project manager receives delegated authority from the sponsor and in turn delegates tasks to the team members. It is best for the project manager to have enough knowledge of the technical area to know when they are being misled but they do not need to be experts—they have team members to provide that expertise. Moreover, if they are experts, they find it hard to resist micromanaging, when they should be managing the whole project.

From this, we begin to identify which skills the project manager really does need. Why not ask them? I have recently seen unpublished interim results from a survey of project managers, across all industries, which can be distilled as follows:

Most challenging overall factor: People
Overall factor with the biggest impact on success: People
Most critical specific factor: Team motivation and ownership
Most challenging task: Getting real commitment to targets
Most difficult type of person: Uncommitted, unwilling to take responsibility

Keeping multitudinous IT systems up to date is not seen as critical to success but getting people to do what you want is. This is a skill that can be imparted with training. Yet, I have experience of a large clinical research organization, with project managers responsible for budgets of up to US $20 million each, where they had received no training at all in the type of skills that we are discussing here. They were however trained to the hilt on the IT systems. I will just for the present say that negotiation, communication, and problem analysis come near the top of my list of essential project manager skills.

Consistent Planning

The structure for protocol development in Figure 7 is typical of procedures in common use in the pharmaceutical industry. It complies with good clinical practice (GCP) and, assuming all the correct data are passed down the line, would be expected to generate a workable protocol. The reason this is not always the case is its unidirectional design. A list of requirements at the outset is unlikely to be complete and unless this list is challenged by the recipient, gaps may remain unfilled, or even worse, be filled by guesswork. A more secure system is shown in Figure 11, which I use for all types of clinical-trial-related work. The essence is that at both the functional requirements stage (what the client wants from the project) and at the selection of methodology stage, two-way communication with the client is the rule. Tools that help this process are largely already available, in the form of standard operating procedurest (SOPs) to check feasibility and as databases of information on how methods performed in the past, to name but two. A project manager with a good grasp of this process should be able to define any project within his span of technical knowledge as long as he is empowered by top management to carry out the negotiations required. Projects too often fail when this empowerment has not been carried out (such as the "project coordinator").

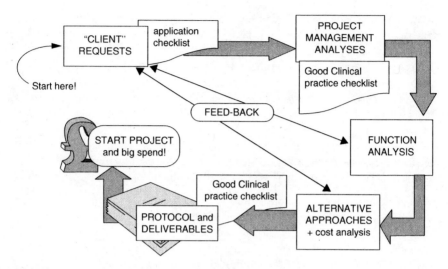

Figure 11 Clinical trials definition process. *Source*: Courtesy of Centre for Medicines Research International, Epsom, UK. R&D e-Factbook, 2007.

Precisely the same process can be used at any level in clinical research, whether one is planning a single study or a whole clinical development program. In practice, within pharmaceutical companies, the latter more often resembles Figure 7 probably because at this stage much less is clear about the whole drug project. For single studies, the trap to avoid is using tried and tested methods on a production line basis. This can stifle creativity.

I am making this point about defining projects because it is a key function of the project manager. It is often seen as a mechanistic process but it is actually subject to organization and culture. This is because to make it work the project manager has to be good with people—to negotiate effectively and to identify what drives them. One of the many problems we have is that pharmaceutical companies are often dominated by prestigious scientists, mostly recruited because of their reputations in research and medicine, so the project manager needs to negotiate with them with sensitivity and intelligence.

Communications

I used to err on the side of overcommunication but I am beginning to reconsider that. Something that has triggered the change of heart is that if I am away from my desk for an hour I can have 20 e-mails by the time I get back. A good communication plan is essential for any project and I have had to start saying to people, "Do not use me as the project postman." If I have delegated a task, there is no need to send the deliverable via me, it can go directly but just tell me it has happened. I will decide if I want to verify it. So, I have come round to the view that the communication plan should state clearly what not to do as well as what to do. That is something on which the project managers can put their own personal stamp.

Integrating Project Management

I have already expressed a degree of dismay at how the project manager's role can be so easily misunderstood. By now, I was expecting that clinical research would have closed the competence gap with other industries but there is still some distance between them and us. This often seems to be related to a perception that project management is a noncore discipline, a kind of additional layer or rather optional or peripheral activity. For example, one fast growing pharmaceutical company spent huge effort (and money) on developing a wide range of new processes for managing clinical trials but omitted even to think about any consistent approach to project planning. For the very few trials that did have some kind of plan, they could not be handed over between managers as nobody understood anyone else's plan.

This again is a problem related to culture. If the project manager lacks empowerment, it seems unlikely that there will be much investment in tools for their job. Clinical trials by definition are projects and their management as such must be a core activity. This means that all other existing (and usually highly effective) systems and processes must be integrated into the project-orientated culture. If this were happening, we should be seeing that every organization conducting clinical trials would have among its SOPs one for project management. Otherwise, how could consistency prevail? I do not think I need to set out what such an SOP should contain. Essentially, anyone who knows what project management is, and is experienced in clinical research, should be able to write it. But many organizations do not have it and some that say they do actually misunderstand it. I have seen a "project management" SOP that makes no mention whatever of any of the key elements that I have been considering here but instead concerns itself with GCP compliance and related issues. Study management is not project management.

I agonized earlier about the fragmentation of computer systems and we have the same problem with the way some companies think about managing clinical trials. We should be integrating everything we do by using the project plan as the catalyst for action, not as something we suddenly remember to do when we have got everything else set up. There are extremely simple things we can do to achieve this. We can embed in our plans dynamic links to our SOPs so that the standard to which a task has to be carried out is inseparable from the task itself. We can insert the key quality stages in the plan so that the quality system is no longer yet another independent layer for us to manage. From another direction, we can embed the baseline project plan in our project-specific procedures as an appendix that will help to control slippage by reminding everyone of what we originally planned to do.

Getting Things Done—The Clinical Project Manager's Authority

At several stages in this chapter the project manager's vital need for top management support has been emphasized. If this one need were satisfied, many companies, which are now average performers, would be among the leaders in their fields.

How to Create Empowerment

Even if one's own scenario seems so disappointing, there is hope! If many of the causes of project failure are related to poor communications, the project manager can achieve much by ensuring that what has been agreed is widely known within the organization, especially in the upper strata. When a clinical plan or protocol has been agreed, why not send a summary to top management itemizing the key deliverables, who is responsible for them, and when they have been promised? Even if top management does nothing, is it more or less likely that drug supply (for example) will be on time and correctly packaged when the pharmacy department knows who is aware of the agreement? Eventually of course, top management starts to take some notice of these succinct summaries from clinical research, especially when they are followed by positive progress reports.

At the beginning of the section "People in Projects," I drew attention to getting the balance right when communicating to senior management. This is what I have just been talking about here. The principle is that busy managers are not going to read long reports but they do need key information regularly. You do not want a director complaining to your line manager that you have not been keeping them updated.

Clinical Research in the New Global Village

Eleven years ago, I speculated on a few of the many factors influencing the world of clinical research. As noted earlier here, the development of information technology has had a heavy impact. At the time, I was expecting to see major improvements in planning, stemming from key areas such as collecting information to produce estimates of time scale, cost, and labor. Today, CROs are especially adept at this, and they build up quotations from complex matrices comprising items of effort. But, assumptions are sometimes too simplistic, for example, the assumption that the effort will be applied flat across the duration of a task (or for the project manager across the whole project). My impression is that clinical trials are more heavily front loaded than other types of project, related inter alia to the need for external approvals to start work, so planning effort on a flat basis is not going to work. So that although quite extensive and sophisticated databases of cost information are increasingly available, they still need intelligent application.

Cracking the Patient Supply Problem

One of the most significant developments of the last decade has been the emergence of site management organizations (SMOs). This was the response to the need for

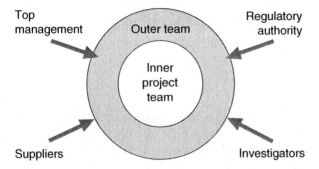

Top
management

Regulatory
authority

Suppliers

Investigators

Figure 12 Who is in a project team? Example participants. *Source*: Courtesy of Centre for Medicines Research International, Epsom, UK. R&D e-Factbook, 2007.

much closer involvement of investigator sites with clinical trials and has a close fit with the need to bring investigators nearer to the core team. Figure 12 illustrates the principle with some examples of the types of people and organizations contributing to project success. We have already considered the problem of delegating control to people remote from the core team and SMOs have the potential to mitigate this.

Yet SMOs do not dominate the clinical trials landscape while another major trend has emerged in recent years. This is the migration of studies eastwards, first to central and then eastern Europe and now to Asia. Initially, cost was the main driver but now access to drug-naïve patients seems to be the main reason. Clearly, dispersing trials ever wider across the globe, with attendant communication and cultural challenges, will impact on project planning and control. In my experience, relatively mundane factors such as time zones can have disproportionately adverse effects on project control. They do of course need to be addressed at the planning stage, particularly when defining communication standards.

A disappointment, especially in the United Kingdom, has been the slow development of interfaces with National Health Service medical records. This presented the opportunity to obtain very reliable estimates of eligible patients but most secondary-care-based studies still largely rely on informal estimates from investigators—which always have to be downgraded for realism.

Good Idea—But Will It Work?

CROs again have been pioneers in another planning technique, that of feasibility studies. I noted in 1996 how underused this was then, and that still is the case, but at least some effort is being made now in a few places. However, it seems again to focus mostly on patient recruitment whereas key bottlenecks such as slow local regulatory approvals could kill a study in a particular country. Curiously, trial simulation using proprietary software seems to be rarely used despite its promise. My guess is that because pharmaceutical companies persist in compressing planning time unrealistically, they rarely sanction such exercises. However, let us consider when they should be done—not at the planning stage once a study has been approved for startup but at the clinical development plan stage or even earlier. No doubt some companies are doing this but the practice does not seem to be common.

Project Team Integration

As discussed earlier, modern communications have clearly enabled project teams to work more closely together. This is related to no small extent to the visibility of success. There is no greater motivator than success itself (6) and with cycle times for many tasks now much shorter, most people can see results every day. Not only that, communication should expose them to the wider scope of the project; even if the results are not your own, seeing success somewhere else concentrates the mind. Dedicated study Web sites are being used but mainly as information repositories not as motivators. In the first edition of this book, I proposed the "virtual team territory" as a way of building more team involvement. It may or may not have been a good idea at the time but today Web surfing is a normal activity for just about all of us. A project Web site that is interesting would not have to drive people towards it, yet, study newsletters are still being sent out on paper.

The Future Is Today

Well, almost. Such is the pace of change that the future tends to be here before we have had time to prepare for it. However, what strikes me about clinical trials is the conflict between the breakneck speed with which some changes occur and the lack of progress in others. For the latter, I am particularly conscious of organizational and cultural models for managing trials. Throughout this chapter, I have frequently drawn comparisons between pharmaceutical companies and others that run projects. I have just been looking at 20 advertisements for clinical project manager and director positions. Not a single one demands a professional qualification or membership in project management or even a record of having received training in it. They all require formal training in GCP. They do require experience in project management but that does not necessarily imply competence (because it may not be practiced to a high standard). If you look at equivalent positions in say engineering, you will be lucky to be shortlisted for an interview without at least a membership and more likely certification by examination such as Project Management Professional or PRINCE2 practitioner. This surely is a measure of how seriously our industry takes the discipline. It is not simply a matter of not weighting project management sufficiently per se; it is a misconception as to what it is. This final section is really about what makes a project manager successful and it is not a solely mechanistic practice. Systems do not manage projects, people do, and they must have the skills and aptitudes to do it. Training people to use Primavera, Concerto, or Microsoft Project does not make them a project manager.

Keeping It Simple

This last fallacy causes more damage than you might think. It is very easy to be highly impressed by the software salesperson's patter such that your organization invests heavily in a complex system that promises to solve all your project problems. Of course, it is not going to and you end up with a massive training overhead and most likely a partial implementation because the whole undertaking is too complex. Advanced concepts such as Critical Chain Method (7) have great potential but this is unlikely to be realized if the project managers are not trained in what project management is. This is not fiction—I have seen it happen. So the message here is, if you cannot invest in fully training your project managers, use simple systems well rather than complex things badly. Any company that fully implements classical project management, i.e., Gantt and PERT methods, will easily put itself ahead of the game without feeling the need for the latest cutting edge methodologies.

EDC's Birthright Undervalued?

I really did expect that EDC would have dominated clinical trials by now. This was not just because of its potential to improve data quality and to shorten the data management process but also (and probably more so) as a tool for better collaboration and project control. Today's perception of EDC seems to be heavily toward the former benefits with very little towards the latter. There are now a huge number of EDC vendors because basically the technology is not difficult. What is far more challenging is getting the best out of the technology. Surely there is a connection between a general lack of realization of project management best practice and this misunderstanding of what EDC could bring to it. Thus, these many vendors mostly offer stand-alone EDC systems or services that are not integrated into management systems. Surely EDC should solve one of our most pressing problems—keeping control of progress. That function does however appear to be addressed by IVRS in some of its guises, although that was not conceived for the purpose originally.

Cash Is King

Some readers will probably be surprised that I have not so far mentioned cost management to a significant extent. This is because among the three classical targets of time, cost, and deliverables, cost is relatively straightforward to manage, but more importantly, it is less critical to project success than is time. Put simply, it is better to overspend and be on time than to be late and on budget. I did protest earlier against the proliferation of spreadsheets for progress tracking; the same has happened with budgets. We are now increasingly seeing the use of trial management systems that manage a part of the budget, but not all of it, so that spreadsheets have to be used to fill the gaps. I do not see this as changing rapidly in the near future. It is worth remembering that a major part of the budget is staff time and many drug companies do not bother to track this. CROs, of course, are usually much better at it. I do believe that controlling human resource deployment on projects is a vastly underused tool and many top managers would be shocked at how much they are wasting, if they ever looked at it. I mentioned above the use of the Critical Chain Method and importantly this prioritizes resource as the major constraint to manage. Very oddly, I know of a company that has implemented a Critical Chain based system but without the resource module, which, of course, largely emasculates it. There is clearly an understanding gap at senior level. In addition, there is a training gap at project level, with managers quite often lacking appreciation of the basics of accounting.

The Born-Again Project Manager

The new style of manager will need to be highly analytical, tenacious, and an excellent negotiator. They will need to understand finance and contracts at a familiarization level—even if the company has a specialist contracts department. After all, only the project manager knows what the internal client wants in enough detail. They will not need to be technical specialists but will need enough scientific knowledge to be able to evaluate information. They will need to know where to get experts when they need them. To meet these and many other challenges, the project manager needs a certain skill set that top management needs to make available. At the same time, top management needs to be much clearer as to its own role or "empowerment" will never be anything more than jargon. The future clinical project manager will need

- more authority,
- more status and recognition compared with line management,
- better people skills, for example, negotiation and leadership,
- more support from project sponsors, and
- an operating environment structured for successful projects.

A Visible Means of Support

The last item above yet again seems to mark out clinical trials from other projects in general. It is not common to see the proper implementation of a particular component that is generally considered elsewhere to be a part of best practice. This is the project office that provides administrative support to the project manager. Its purpose is to relieve them of much of the routine work such as maintaining libraries of planning templates and progress report formats, maybe maintaining the project Web site, and collecting progress information. A few companies are starting to implement this at study level but it is by no means the norm. If it becomes common currency, it will indicate at last a commitment to best practice and an appreciation at senior level of what project management is.

SO IS CLINICAL PROJECT MANAGEMENT FIT FOR PURPOSE?

We have seen that there is a wide variation between companies in terms of drug development performance. This suggests a wide variation in capability for all components of drug development with, as we know, clinical trials making a very major contribution to that. Fully implemented, simple and basic project management can make dramatic improvements but the main gap seems to be not so much in systems as in culture and organization. Changing behaviors is the most difficult thing we can do but we have to do it.

REFERENCES

1. CMR International. R&D e-Factbook, CMR International, Epsom, UK, 2007.
2. PRINCE2. Office of Government Commerce, Norwich, UK. Available at http://www. ogc.gov.uk/methods_prince_2.asp.
3. APM Body of Knowledge. 5th edn. Association for Project Management, High Wycombe, UK, 2006.
4. Curry S, Brown R. The target product profile as a planning tool in drug discovery research. Business Briefing. Pharmatech, London, UK, 2003. Available at http://www. touchbriefings.com/cdps/cditem.cfm?nid=17&cid=5. Accessed on August 24, 2007.
5. Expert Group on Phase One Clinical Trials: Final report. The Stationery Office. December 7, 2006. Available at http://www.dh.gov.uk/en/Publicationsandstatistics/ Publications/PublicationsPolicyAndGuidance/DH_063117.
6. Maslow A. A theory of human motivation. Psychol Rev 1943;50:370–396.
7. North River Press, Great Barrington, USA, 1997.

7

Regulatory Project Management

Nicholas Wells
Independent Pharma Consultants, Kent, U.K.

INTRODUCTION

Regulatory affairs (RA) over the last two decades has played an ever-increasing role in the development of new medicinal products with the average development program, from inception of an idea through to market, taking between 12 to 15 years. The estimated expenditure by pharmaceutical companies over this period and before any cost can be recovered is currently between $500 (£350) million and $800 (£500) million for a new chemical entity.

For a medicine to be used by patients, the identified candidate product must be tested for quality, safety, and efficacy and then assessed and authorized by the Ministry of Health (MOH) or a regulatory agency. Thus, with the complexity and number of pharmaceutical regulations increasing, the role of the RA professional has become pivotal to the success of a new product and ultimately the company.

Figure 1 illustrates a typical example of the steps involved in a development program during which the RA professional must use his/her skills to guide the project team through the maze of regulations.

Once a marketing authorization application has been approved and a license granted, the regulatory professional's role does not stop there. There are many maintenance activities to ensure the product remains on the market and in compliance with any new regulations, (e.g., patient information leaflet (PIL) user testing and Braille requirements for packaging). The RA department is involved to the end of the product life cycle either to divest the product and transfer the ownership of the license to a third party or to cancel the marketing authorization. Figure 2 illustrates a standard product life cycle.

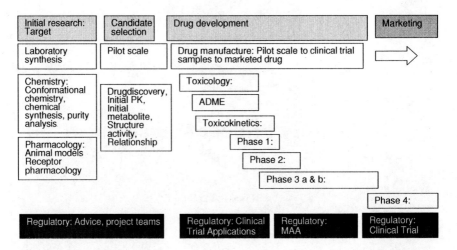

Figure 1 Drug development from inception to market—the role of regulatory affairs. *Abbreviations*: PK, pharmacokinetics; ADME, absorption, drug metabolism, and excretion; MAA, marketing authorization application.

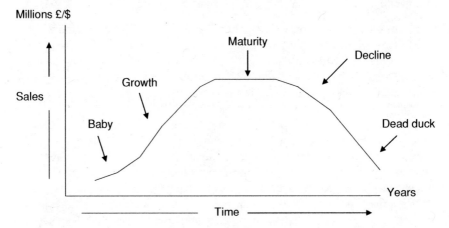

Figure 2 A standard product life cycle—product X.

For many years, each national health authority developed its own specific regulations, assessment time lines, and processes for assessing and approving license applications in isolation from each other. The result of this was a very broad and diverse list of regulations and processes throughout the world.

In the 1990s, the International Conference on Harmonisation (ICH) was initiated to review, develop, and make recommendations for harmonized guidelines. The broad areas for review included guidance for establishing efficacy, safety, and manufacturing control of a medicine for public use.

ICH is comprised of representatives from the following:

- European Federation of Pharmaceutical Industries Association (EFPIA)
- European Commission
- Japanese Pharmaceutical Manufacturers Association (JPMA)
- U.S. Food and Drug Administration
- Pharmaceutical Research and Manufacturers of America (PhRMA)
- Japanese Ministry of Health

From the established guidelines, draft guidelines, and position papers, the RA professional is able to advise senior management and also the global core project team (GCPT) on current regulatory requirements. However, it must be remembered that these are guidelines and the regulatory professional must interpret them and advise on how best to comply with them or present an argument to the regulatory authorities if the data is not available to support a particular directive or regulation. The regulatory professional, throughout the development of a new product, is part of a multidisciplinary team and this can be at the corporate, regional, or national level.

What Is Project Management?

A project is a fixed task and, as in the case of a new product development project lasting many years, will have many smaller defined projects throughout the development and life cycle. Broadly speaking, a project has a starting point and a definitive end point.

Project management is the application of knowledge, skills, tools, and techniques to a broad range of activities in order to meet the requirements of the particular project. Project management knowledge and practices are best described in terms of their component processes. These processes can be placed into five process groups:

- Initiating
- Planning
- Executing
- Controlling
- Closing

Thus, within RA there are numerous types of subprojects that support the higher-level project of developing, registering, and maintaining the product and finally divesting or canceling the product license.

Working effectively within project teams is extremely important for the successful outcome of any project, whether it is a major new chemical entity submission or a manufacturing compliance problem requiring a number of variations to be submitted to resolve the issue. This may seem obvious to the reader but anyone who has worked in a team may appreciate the difficulties that may arise due to conflicting resources, time, budgets, and workload.

The typical skills required by any project team member are as follows:

Global Product Marketing Plan

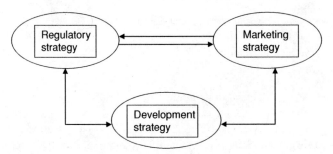

Figure 3 Global product marketing plan.

- knowledge and expertise in their field,
- listening and communication skills,
- pragmatic and analytical skills,
- problem solving, and
- proactive, "can do" attitude.

Examples of regulatory activities/projects:

- New drug applications (NDA)/marketing authorization applications (MAA)
- Investigational NDA/clinical trial applications
- License renewals, license variations
- Product divestment (change of ownership) and acquisition due diligence
- Review of promotional material
- Regulatory intelligence
- Crisis management—product recalls and so on

REPORTING TO THE GCPT

The GCPT is a multifunctional team responsible for the strategic management of a pharmaceutical product or a group of products in a therapeutic area. Team members are collectively responsible for the development of a new product, the global submission plan (for clinical trial applications, MAA, and any postapproval variation applications), any postapproval commitments, and general maintenance of the life cycle of the product. Ultimately, the global product marketing plan is developed (Fig. 3).

The role of the GCPT RA team member(s) is one of advice, guidance, and direction on the current regulations and best practices that relates to the development of the product. The regulatory member of the GCPT is a senior member of the regulatory department, normally a regulatory professional with several years' experience of regulatory submissions and detailed therapeutic product knowledge. Regulatory job titles vary from one company to the next but usually the experience

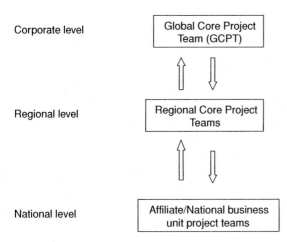

Corporate level   Global Core Project Team (GCPT)

Regional level   Regional Core Project Teams

National level   Affiliate/National business unit project teams

Figure 4 Information flow from and to the global core project team.

required would match a regulatory title of a senior manager or an associate director or director.

To enable the GCPT RA representative to provide up-to-date and accurate information to the GCPT, the GCPT RA lead relies on his/her experience and the expertise of the regulatory subteam members for regional and RA area representative knowledge. An example of this could be advice on the current regional or national regulatory assessment and approval times for clinical trial applications and MAA. It is useful to be aware of the statutory regulatory assessment times but vitally important to be aware of "real" pickup and assessment times at the national MOH or regulatory authorities. These "real" assessment times may be longer than the statutory time lines due to the MOH or agency workload being greater than available resources. The information flow from and to the GCPT can vary in different companies but, generally, the flow is as described in Figure 4.

Global Core Project

The GCPT has the responsibility of developing a new product through the development phases to registration and then general postregistration life cycle activities. The GCPT may be comprised of team members from other departments such as marketing, manufacturing, medical affairs, clinical research, and RA. The GCPT makes decisions based on the company objective, therapeutic and marketing considerations, and on regulatory information collected from the subteams. The GCPT takes an overview of the project by setting ambitious but realistic milestones, determining rate-limiting steps, and monitoring progress.

RA Subteam

The RA subteam is generally comprised of the GCPT representative who leads the RA subteam and the regional leads—EU, Japan, Chemistry, Manufacturing and Controls (CMC), United States, and project management.

Regional area leads review all aspects of the regional legislation and coordinate the information gathered from the national or affiliate RA experts. They then present the regional consensus through to the core project team RA lead. The regional team is responsible for implementing the project milestones for its region and facilitates and monitors the progress of the project with the local national affiliates liaising upwards to the GCPT RA lead and keeping them informed of the progress.

Other RA Support to RA Subteams

Senior RA management with regional or local RA expertise is available on a consultancy basis for the RA subteam. Other departments responsible for promotion, company core data sheets, RA operations, regulatory intelligence, and other external representatives may all at some point contribute to the RA subteam.

National (Affiliate) RA Country Expert

Like the regional area project lead, the country expert looks at the project from a national basis and feeds up the national requirements and/or concerns through to the regional RA subteam lead. In some pharmaceutical companies, the regional RA department or national affiliate RA departments make the regulatory submissions and liaise with their regulatory agencies. However, increasingly with electronic submission a separate publishing group within the global RA (GRA) group is responsible for producing and submitting applications to regional and/or national regulatory agencies.

Once regulatory approval has been received, the local affiliates or business units are responsible for launching the new product onto their respective markets with the GCPT taking an overview of the global submission plan.

Additionally, at the national level, small business unit teams may be formed to develop a product or a group of products postapproval. This team is comprised of regulatory, marketing, medical affairs, medical information, clinical research, and external advertising or PR companies.

Meeting Frequency

All project teams whether the GCPT, RA subteam, or the affiliate business unit team meet on a regular basis—from once a week to once a month and may, on occasions, if warranted, meet more frequently. The ultimate aim is to ensure that the product project plan—whether a development plan working towards first registration or a postregistration project plan to maintain or increase the market share of the product—is followed and amended as appropriate.

GCPT RA Responsibilities

The regulatory therapeutic lead is the primary interface between the GRA department and the GCPT. The GCPT RA lead is a fully qualified regulatory professional capable of representing the GRA department and competently speaking on other RA areas. Their main functions include the following:

- They develop and own global consistent high-quality product strategy informed by deep therapeutic knowledge. They
  - are responsible for the key agency-specific inputs into the strategy (development and marketed products).
  - obtain input and approval from the associated areas and other regulatory functions.
  - maintain deep therapeutic expertise to inform on formal and informal RA guidance.

The GCPT RA lead routinely attends the GCPT meetings and may invite other subteam members to participate on an ad hoc basis. The GCPT RA lead should always be aware of the interactions between GCPT members and other functions within the RA department, for example, with the team responsible for CMC.

The GCPT RA representative also leads the RA subteam and this is a very time-consuming role for the GCPT RA lead. However, all communications providing updates to all team members are vital for keeping the project teams on task. The main functions include the following:

- They serve as a single GCPT representative and maintain overall RA project responsibility. They
  - attend GCPT meetings as a single RA representative and represent RA to senior management.
  - maintain communication of RA subteam project activities to the GCPT and from the GCPT to RA subteams.
  - assure alignment of development and regulatory strategies.
  - are responsible for the content at key agency interactions and participation at meetings.
  - manage RA response to crisis situations.
  - facilitate prioritization, resources, and planning in the GCPT.

The GCPT RA lead is the owner of the regulatory strategy and is responsible for the content and completion of the regulatory strategy for the product. The GCPT RA lead is also responsible for any major agency-specific aspects of the regulatory strategy (e.g., an agency rejection of a particular end point) and has to defend the regulatory strategy to the GCPT and senior management.

The end product of the regulatory strategy is meeting the regulatory objectives for submissions to the European Medicines Agency (EMEA), FDA, and other agencies while maintaining the perspective on safety and efficacy required for approval and long-term management of the product.

The GCPT RA lead is also responsible for the description of anticipated indications as well as anticipated hurdles to approval and for reflecting an understanding of competitive products and historical agency behavior. Their functions also include the following:

- They oversee filing content and strategy. They
  - prepare and own the broad dossier design.
  - are responsible for clinical trial applications and support of clinical trials with input from departmental sections and RA subteams.
  - keep marketed products in compliance and on the market.
  - are responsible for review and approval of global company core data sheets or for advertising and promotion.
  - develop and maintain deep relationships with key health agencies.

REGULATORY ACTIVITIES DURING THE PRODUCT'S LIFE

Discovery/Nonclinical

Early development of a product entails the toxicological studies to develop an understanding of the safety profile for the product. Early development is where potential products are screened using minimal animal models to establish the basic pharmacokinetic and the initial pharmacological results. The project team may be looking for products with a longer duration of activity, an increased rate of absorption, reduced or increased peak concentration, improved safety profile (reduced side effects), and a favorable response to a pharmacological model with minimal toxicity.

The regulatory project team members can advise on the current legislation to the type and number of species to be used for a toxicity program and the type and duration of studies.

The reported data from the nonclinical studies are then collated and the regulatory team begins to compile the nonclinical section of the Investigational Medicinal Product Dossier, which is the scientific information for a clinical trial application. The nonclinical data also form the basis of the nonclinical section and summaries of the marketing application (NDA/MAA).

Types of Studies

- General toxicology studies
  - Acute, subchronic, and chronic toxicity tests are conducted to determine the effect of a new product on the health and mortality during various lengths of exposure, such as, single-dose study and repeat-dose studies spanning over a number of weeks and months, for example, 1, 2, and 4 weeks; 3, 6, 9, 12, and 24 months.

- Reproductive toxicology studies
  - ○ Developmental toxicity tests (teratogenicity) are designed to evaluate the capacity of the new product to cause abnormalities in the embryo and fetus.
  - ○ Reproductive toxicity tests are designed to study the effects of the new product on fertility and fecundity.
- Mutagenicity and carcinogenicity studies
  - ○ These types of studies are designed to examine the potential of the new product to cause benign or malignant tumors.
- ADME—Absorption, drug metabolism, and excretion studies.
- Toxicokinetic studies.

Clinical

From Figure 1, you can see that the regulatory input is throughout the development program and as the product nears registration, the involvement of the regulatory team member in all project teams becomes increasingly important.

The clinical development program is an area where the regulatory team member is crucial to help the project team understand the individual country requirements and time lines for approval.

Many situations can occur that require the regulatory team member to liaise with the GCPT and the regulatory subteam at the regional and local level. For example, if a study drug is being compared to an existing marketed drug, termed a "comparator drug," then the regulatory team member has to be aware of the registration status in all countries where that comparator drug is to be used in the trial. If a country does not have the comparator registered then that product may be considered as an investigational product and additional information may be required to support its use in a clinical trial. Table 1 discusses the various phases involved in clinical development (Fig. 5).

Submission

The role of GCPT RA lead in the submission of any application varies at different stages (Table 2). Below is an example of a major submission such as an NDA or an MAA.

Approval and Launch

Prior to the approval of a new product by the MOH or regulatory authorities, the GCPT along with RA regional or national leads and their respective marketing groups plan the launch of the product to the market. This needs to be achieved as soon as possible after the regulatory approval has been received.

To launch a product on to the market, a consideration is required on the timing of the production of the product, its packaging, storage, and delivery to wholesalers and pharmacies. This includes the design and approval of the

Table 1 Phases of Clinical Development

Phase	Phase 1	Phase 2	Phase 3a	Phase 3b	Phase 4
Number of subjects	Up to 20 or 30	Up to 100	100–1000	100–1000	>1000
Type of subjects	Healthy volunteers	Selected patients	Patients	Patients	Patients
Principal purpose	Dose finding	Dose ranging and confirming	Efficacy of chosen dose	Comparison with existing treatments	General postmarketing experience of the drug
Safety	Acute tolerability	Detailed safety assessments	General safety monitoring	General safety monitoring	General safety monitoring
Where usually conducted	Specialist units	Specialized hospital centers	General hospital centers	General hospitals (and general practice)	General hospitals (and general practice)

Phases of Clinical Development (ICH E8)

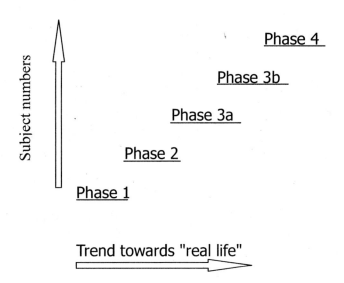

Figure 5 Phases of clinical development (ICH E8). *Abbreviation*: ICH, International Conference on Harmonisation.

packaging and patient information leaflet. The summary of product characteristics (SmPC) must be approved and printed for use by the company sales representative.

Promotional materials require internal approval by marketing, medical affairs, and RA teams prior to use. The RA team is involved as a support and can approve from a regulatory standpoint but the responsibility of the "launch" is ultimately a regional or national marketing function.

Postapproval

Regulatory involvement in the life cycle management of a product is concerned with the postapproval development of a product to maintain the product on the market and also to support the product's market share; it involves

- variations,
- pharmacovigilance,
- manufacture and distribution,
- working with the marketing team to facilitate business objectives, and
- line extensions (Table 3).

Life cycle management involves all three levels of the product development teams, i.e., the GCPT, the regional project team, and the national business unit teams.

Table 2 GCPT RA Lead Roles and Responsibilities in Completing a Major Submission

Activity	RA function	Responsibility
Resource planning	GCPT RA lead	Responsible
	Regulatory operations	Support
	CMC	Support
	RA area	Inform
	RA management	Approve
Document list	GCPT RA lead	Responsible
	Regulatory operations	Inform
	CMC	Support
	RA area	Approve
	RA management	Inform
RA review and input	GCPT RA lead	Approve and support
	Regulatory operations	None
	CMC	Approve and support
	RA area	Support
	RA management	Responsible
Peer review	GCPT RA lead	Responsible
	Regulatory operations	Support
	CMC	Support
	RA area	Inform
	RA management	Support
Collect documents and assemble submission	GCPT RA lead	Support
	Regulatory operations	Support
	CMC	Support
	RA area	Responsible
	RA management	Inform
Sign off	GCPT RA lead	Support
	Regulatory operations	Responsible
	CMC	Approve and support
	RA area	Approve and support
	RA management	Inform
Ship	GCPT RA lead	None
	Regulatory operations	Responsible
	CMC	Inform
	RA area	Inform
	RA management	None

Abbreviations: GCPT, global core project team; RA, regulatory affairs; CMC.

Table 3 Regulatory and Marketing Life Cycle Management Strategy—Line Extensions

Regulatory strategy	Marketing strategy
New chemical/salt	How will it be marketed? • Own marketing • Copromotion • Comarketing
New dosage form New delivery system	What will be the price? • How to get a higher price?
New route of administration	Will brand names be the same?
New indication	What will happen globally/nationally?
New patient population	What is the strategy for further line extensions?

Throughout the life cycle of a product, there will be positive influences and negative influences or events that will impact the success of a product. These influences can be both regulatory and commercial (Table 4). In either case, the regulatory professional has to work effectively in a team using his/her knowledge and influencing skills to facilitate a successful outcome.

TIMELY PROVISION OF QUALITY REGULATORY INFORMATION OR DOCUMENTATION

Quality systems are paramount in today's regulatory environment. The key is to establish a simple and user-friendly system as it will help with compliance.

Definition

"A quality system to ensure that users of medicinal products, the applicants, the regulators are satisfied with scientific advice, opinions, the establishment of MRLs, inspection and assessment reports and related documents, taking into consideration legal requirements and guidance in order to protect and promote human and animal health"
Source: EMEA. October 16, 2000. Doc ref: EMEA/D/30342/00/QM/IA

To establish a quality system in RA, it is necessary to write and maintain a series of standard operating procedures (SOPs) to ensure the regulatory operations are comprehensive and current.

SOPs are the first port of call for any inspector when carrying out routine periodic inspections. However, SOPs should not be so prescriptive that they cause

Table 4 Examples of Positive and Negative Regulatory and Commercial
Influences on a Product Life Cycle

Positive influences	
Regulatory	Commercial
Patent protection • initial and supplementary	Combined products
Data protection	Modified new active substance • pro drugs • metabolites • racemates
Line extensions	Licensing deals
Competitor restrictions	Competitor failure Reclassification from POM to OTC
Negative influences	
Regulatory	Commercial
Product recalls Safety • Epidemiology • Restrictions • Warnings	International Regulatory Agencies Formularies Competitors Parallel imports
Competitor restrictions	Generics • New active substance • Biotechnology
SmPC harmonization	OTC competitors

Abbreviations: POM, prescription only medicine; OTC, over the counter SmPC, summary of product characteristics.

noncompliance as this would require a deviation record to be compiled and, after a number of reports, a process review.

Regulatory SOPs should cross refer to any relevant corporate SOPs and be published on an Intranet Web site. SOPs require frequent review to ensure that current practices and improvements are reflected.

Wherever appropriate, regulatory process should be reviewed and adapted to ensure a culture of continuous improvement. Process maps are useful to establish working patterns and resources and can form a part of the regulatory training.

Document Quality

As regulatory professionals, we are expected to provide high quality and accurate information. To this end, the RA professional can utilize various resources, for example, the ICH guidelines outline the requirements for establishing and reporting the safety, efficacy, and quality of a product. Many countries outside now refer to the ICH guidelines for product registrations in their countries or cross refer to specific competent authority assessments of a drug MAA. Additionally, the EMEA Web site has a clear guidance on how applications of all types should be structured. Under ICH, the common technical document (CTD) is a prescribed format that clearly outlines the structure for a marketing authorization and the submissions using an electronic CTD (eCTD) format also have a clear guidance.

The EMEA quality review documents or templates provide a clear guidance on the structure and content of the SmPC and not following this guidance will cause delays in the assessment of any applications involving the submission of a new or updated SmPC.

The regulatory professional is responsible for ensuring that the language in any application is clear and accurate and that the language used does not lead to misinterpretation by the assessors. The aim is to prevent or at least reduce the number of potential questions from the assessor and an unclear ambiguous content will lead to many questions (or a request for further information).

Timely Submissions and Approval

The regulatory professional needs to be aware of the current timelines for assessment and approvals of all types of regulatory submissions, including clinical trial application (CTA) submissions, variations and renewals, and MAA. They should not only be aware of the statutory assessment times but also the "real" assessment times. This is because regulatory agencies also need to manage their workload and, as a result, the time taken in picking up and validating applications may vary due to the agency workload. Regulatory agencies may invalidate applications based on quality issues and incomplete supporting documentation.

Regulatory Information and Records Management

Good document management and product history is vital to the regulatory professional. How this information is managed and recorded can save many hours searching through dusty old submissions. Depending on the size and available resources of a company, document management systems such as "documentum" can be employed. For smaller companies with limited resources, a well-designed folder structure can be beneficial so long as it is maintained and used consistently by appropriately trained users.

ESTABLISHING THE IMPORTANCE OF GOOD REGULATORY PRACTICE

What Is Good Regulatory Practice?

Good Regulatory Practice (GRP) can also be described as the best practice. It is the practice of compliance with the regulations and science or technology that relates to the product. This can include the following:

- manufacture and control of the product,
- the toxicology safety testing of the product, and
- establishment of the efficacy for the product.

GRP is also the maintenance of accurate information relating to the license details of the product; thus, it is the continuous review of the national and regional regulations and how they are implemented into quality systems. The principles that can be applied to GRP are as follows:

- Independence
- Accountability
- Transparency
- Confidentiality

The principles that should be applied to the provision of quality documentation are the following:

- Quality documentation supports the safety and efficacy of the finished product by ensuring the quality of the product.
- It outlines all relevant and/or critical parameters.
- It improves the consistency of high-quality reviews.

For example, the objectives of the previously mentioned CTD are to provide a submission of a well-structured document and use of a common format to

- reduce the time and resources needed for compilation,
- facilitate regulatory reviews and communication with the applicant, and
- simplify the exchange of regulatory information between regulatory authorities and between affiliates and subcontractors.

Although this standard format is in place, it should be noted that regulatory agencies experience a number of common deficiencies that effect the assessment of the new product application (Table 5). These deficiencies include an indiscriminate and poorly referenced Quality Overall Summary (QOS), which is something that should be avoided at all costs. The QOS is a key document within the CTD and, when written well, it will instill confidence within the assessor that the rest of the CTD is of an equally high quality.

Considerations for providing a better quality CTD include

- knowing the legislation and guidelines and following recent developments,
- participating in and contributing to the early stages of development,
- making sure that the project team and associated colleagues in the operative functions are aware of the respective regulatory requirements,
- checking all documentation for plausibility or consistency and quality, and
- ensuring that quality is built into the dossier by beginning compilation in the early stages of development.

Table 5 Examples of Common Deficiencies Found in a Common Technical Document

Section of CTD	Common deficiencies
QOS *(within module 2 of the CTD)*	• QOS is indiscriminate • No reference to the current documentation • Missing critical evaluation of the results and cross references to the pages of the documentation • Several experts are named without clear indication of their respective responsibilities
QOS—tables and graphs	• Qualification of experts is not convincing • Required tables and/or graphs are missing • Information provided does not coincide with those supplied in the chemical and pharmaceutical documentation
Chemical and pharmaceutical documentation *(within module 3 of the CTD)*	• Documentation is not structured • Table of contents is missing • Glossary is not submitted • Superfluous documents are submitted • Cross references are not established • Documentation is partially illegible • Name of the preparation is not or rarely identical throughout the documentation • Descriptions of testing methods are repeated several times—cross references are missing

Abbreviations: CTD, common technical document; QOS, quality overall summary.

RA Training

For an effective RA department, a well-developed "continuing professional development" training program is required for all levels of regulatory experience. With pharmaceutical regulations continuously being amended somewhere in the world, being fully informed is important to the success of a product and business.

RA is predominately a degree entry profession but people with the appropriate skills and with internal- and external-industry-led training can become effective regulatory professionals.

To maintain regulatory training, the use of training records can be used to keep a record of internal and external training. Examples of the type of training available to regulatory professionals can be seen in Table 6.

In addition to the technical training courses, the RA professional will also embark on a number of "soft-skills" training courses to aid professional leadership and management development. This will enable them to be effective in their role and include courses and training in

Table 6 Examples of Internal and External Training Available to a Regulatory Professional

Internal training	External training
Regulatory document process training	Courses run by the U.S. RA Professional Society, (RAPS) e.g., the RA certificate
SOP training	Courses run by the EU/International Organization for Professional RA(TOPRA), e.g., the "introductory course," CPD courses, and the MSc in RA
Inspection training	Training courses run by specialized companies such as pharmaceutical RA in the EU and the United States
Internal promotional material awareness training	Some university courses, both in the EU and the United States, now have a RA component. In the United Kingdom, France, and Germany there are specific postgraduate RA courses

Abbreviations: RA, regulatory affairs; SOP, standard operating procedure.

Time management	Budget management
Priority management	Line management
Conflict management	Employment law
Report writing	Communication and presentation
Leadership	PROJECT MANAGEMENT

Conclusion

Bringing a new product through the various stages of product development is a mammoth task, with a huge outlay by the company. Careful project planning at a number of levels, both global and more localized, is essential to ensure that a return on investment can be achieved.

Due to the increasingly important contributory role of RA in these stages of product development, it is vital for regulatory professionals to be suitably skilled. One obvious area that regulatory professionals need to be skilled in is project management but it is equally significant for them to hone skills in other areas such as people, budget, and time management. Training to achieve all of these skills is generally available, both internally and externally.

The production of quality documentation is another area that RA contributes to, not only by hands-on writing, editing, or quality control but also by remaining astutely aware of the latest legislation that can affect this.

In short, RA remains at the center of the planning, running, and execution of any new product development strategy, which highlights the importance of good regulatory project management.

8

Teams

Ralph White
PPMLD Ltd., London, U.K.

Teams—a seemingly innocuous title for a chapter but one that leads us headlong into a fundamental dilemma about the way product development projects are managed. In order to get at the heart of the issue, I will start with a polemic to polarize your thoughts and then build a way to a realistic understanding of pharma product development project teams. This chapter concentrates on teams but will not discuss process tools for planning, scheduling, and budgeting.

THE DILEMMA

Projects rely for success on the cross-functional networking of self-directed experts but most, if not all, pharma companies are organized on vertical management structures of the "command-and-control" variety that has changed little since the industrial revolution. The formal reasons for this are not hard to find. Most people accept that team working is "the right thing to do" but in the world of performance measurement there is scant formal evidence to show that project teams actually improve productivity. However, no one is prepared to risk undertaking the appropriate control experiments (presumably by abolishing teams) because even the most hard-nosed of functional structures have to resort to some form of interface management when dealing with other functions. Most project managers will have proselytized over the years about matrix structures and, with luck, these can progress to become enterprisewide knowledge-sharing networks. In the meantime, they can be little more than a management artifice to encourage a semblance of cross-functional working while reserving the right to control at every level. Too often, that control is exerted in the parochial interest of the line function and not in the interest of the project. Old habits die hard, especially when there is a tendency to appoint managers for their technical acumen rather than their appreciation of product development. In addition, the desirable behavior of a manager as one who supplies subordinates with all the information and resources they need to deliver the task at hand will compete unevenly with the attitude that a manager commands resources and dribbles out information to subordinates on a need-to-know basis. In truth, few pharma project managers feel truly empowered and the matrix is sometimes no more than a goldfish bowl in which their every activity is scrutinized by the holders of resource. Few pharma projects control their own budgets, which, for operational convenience, are held by the functions and so they are viewed with suspicion by project managers from other industries who view budget-holding as the outward symbol of project manager authority. Few traditional managers really understand how a project achieves its objectives; project team behaviors are viewed as vaguely anarchic and certainly bordering on the insubordinate and the time devoted to project team operations can be viewed with suspicion, certainly not to be considered at the annual performance review. This bleak view means that successful project managers need to adopt a wide range of techniques to achieve their objectives and these will also apply equally well when true enterprisewide cultures evolve but we can safely assume that this will not be for some time. I make no apology for this polemic but all is not lost and there are rays of hope. The "T-shaped manager" from BP gives a promising insight into how things could be (1). If teams are redefined as the knowledge-sharing engines of the pharma product development process, then we can see the way forward. In the meantime, this chapter takes a pragmatic approach to the management of teams and should be seen as a checklist of approaches proven to be of value in accumulating knowledge, whatever the organizational culture.

TYPES OF TEAMS

Even the word "team" leads us straight into some difficulty. What does the word team conjure up in your mind? When talking generally about teams, people will often think of a sports team—a U.K. Premier League football team, for instance—a team of highly trained individuals each with a special talent combined into, one hopes, a winning side. Press the question further and you may hear mention of a Special Forces unit of four men—incredibly fit, highly motivated, self-reliant, and dependant upon one another for their very lives. But these are highly specific examples and not general and what comes as more of a surprise is that almost everything we achieve at work and in our social lives involves teams—groups of individuals brought together for a common purpose. There are teams everywhere in pharma and not just the product development ("project") team to which we will be paying most of our attention. Even within a functional department there will be all sorts of ad hoc teams—journal clubs, quality standards, facilities management, techniques groups, "the management team," and even the departmental football team. Teams also permeate all levels of the organization from the functional expert groups ("pharmacokinetics") through to the project team, then to the portfolio team, and up to the main board of the company; all share a commonality in that each is unlikely to be directly managed by one line manager. In fact, to make sense of this diversity, one might define a team as having a "purpose"—a group of individuals with a shared vision of what they need to do and a common understanding of how they can achieve it (2). The corollary is that without a common purpose, the team cannot function.

Within pharmaceutical product development (and we will restrict ourselves to this activity unless otherwise stated), it is quite easy to establish a purpose for a project team—transmute the selected candidate chemical or biological asset into a successful product. So, how do we establish a purpose? The best starting point is to define the target profile. This hybrid defines the eventual product (which could be created from any number of candidates) and allows comparison of the emergent properties of the specific asset under development to ensure it is fit for purpose. The target profile thus helps define the activities involved, the sequence of these activities, and then the required functional membership of the team needed to achieve it. Without too much difficulty, we can list:

- Research champion
- Commercial strategist
- Regulatory professional
- Clinical trials manager
- Nonclinical safety expert
- Chemistry, manufacturing, and controls expert
- Project manager[a]

So far, so good.

This highly skilled team will be colocated, will undertake all the necessary work, and will drive the project to completion—or will it? At this point, the analogy with the teams cited in the opening of this chapter starts seriously to fall apart. Firstly, the purpose is achieved over a number of years: the contribution of these experts fluctuates with the stages of development, with the manufacturing team probably only holding a watching brief during nonclinical development and, conversely, the research champion long gone when the product reaches the market. It is unlikely that team membership will stay the same—people change jobs, take on more responsibilities, leave the company—it may (will) even be punctuated by mergers and acquisitions! Secondly, the work involves very large numbers of people and each of the experts listed above will in turn be reliant on extensive subteams of experts. Thirdly, all involved cannot be physically colocated and may even be in different countries, raising the questions of time, geography, and culture. Finally, we are hostages to the properties of the asset. Unlike working to a set of architects' drawings or engineers' blue print, we know little about the asset at the

---

[a] "Leader, manager, planner, coordinator, facilitator?"—another source of confusion. For our purposes, we will assume that the project manager is a senior-level appointee who is peer to and has the active support of the project sponsors and is able to exert leadership at the strategic level.

outset and there is the ever-present possibility that properties will be revealed at a future date that will bring the project crashing to its knees. Moreover, there are other impediments—the persistence of both a hierarchy ("Do as I say.") and a bureaucracy ("It is the law.") not adapted since the Industrial Revolution can be a significant hindrance to the management of modern self-directing professionals who often have to operate outside the limits of formal authority. Nevertheless, even with these real barriers, it may come as a surprise to know that it is quite possible to define an operating environment within which project teams can thrive and be successful in spite of everything. The longevity and stability of a project team is often overlooked during times of profound organizational change and it is a sad fact that company mergers inevitably start off by bringing together and rationalizing the functional structure (i.e., downsizing) without looking at the collateral damage caused to the project teams.

A BRIEF HISTORY OF PHARMA PROJECT TEAMS

Before defining a successful operating environment for project teams, it is instructive to look briefly at the way these teams have evolved in the industry because examination of their problems helps us to establish some practical ways to manage such teams—*"Those who do not remember the past are destined to repeat it"* (George Santayana).

This has been a rapid evolution. In the not too distant past, the major assumption was that a promising candidate molecule could be transmuted into a successful product by a series of mechanistic steps ("turning the handle"). The maxim was "identify a novel mechanism and the world will beat a path to your door with a clinical application." This worked well for antibiotics but has been unraveled by resistance. It also worked for the first generation of drug receptors but do not forget that the central action of propanolol in the treatment of hypertension was not expected—it was being developed for the treatment of angina through a peripheral effect on cardiac receptors. As the clinical targets have become more elusive and the regulatory and technical barriers have increased, so have the pressures on the project team to perform.

A True Story

Once upon a time, research scientists were working on the three-dimensional structure of hemoglobin and came up with a rational way to chemically modify the tetrameric protein and use it to treat sickle cell disease. The compound was active in the test tube and prevented sickle cells from changing shape when the oxygen levels were reduced. Management chose the candidate for development as an oral life-long treatment for the disease and the research champion, who had no knowledge whatsoever of the drug development process, was appointed the project manager. At the first project team meeting, Pharmacy asked for 5 kg of the compound ("to complete the full scale up to manufacture") and

Chemistry said it would take six months to make ("because that is what we always say"). Toxicology embarked on oral toxicity studies and Metabolism failed to notice that absolute bioavailability was less than 20% because of first pass effects. Toxicology then reported severe gastric irritation; so, the route of administration was changed to intravenous and the safety studies were repeated. The fact that this was to be a chronic therapy was overlooked. During project meetings, a detailed discussion of the finer points of the chemical synthesis would sit side by side with a questioning of why the project was being conducted in the first place. Eventually, a safety package was assembled and it was presented to Clinical Pharmacology, who then said that it was far too dangerous to administer a compound with such a mechanism of action to humans but, after some persuasion, they off-loaded it on to a phase 1 unit at a teaching hospital that was willing to take it on and did not appear to have the same concerns. Meanwhile, clinical management had realized that the resource required to undertake trials in patients was not there and so a heroic "proof-of-concept" study was designed to establish the utility of the compound in the treatment of acute sickle cell crisis. In the event, after a U.S. Investigational New Drug (IND) was granted and clinical trials supplies were manufactured and shipped, the single investigator suddenly lost interest and the project foundered. At the same time, the project manager had approached Commercial Strategy for support, to be asked, "Why are you doing this? There is no market for it!" The project folded, as did the follow-up project, which was looking at an orally acceptable candidate and had already got as far as volunteer studies using a tablet.

This catalogue of horrors gives us useful insight into how projects and, for this particular case, project teams should be organized. But before doing so, there are other more general issues to recall. The first project manager would often be the research champion and the emphasis was to line up the blocks of work needed to complete the registration dossier but without the benefit of a target profile. The process involved "thinking forward," a less polite term is "making it up us you go along." The project teams would evolve in size and it would often be the case that meetings could consist of 40 or 50 individuals discussing subjects ranging from the strategic ("Why are we doing this project?") to the functional ("here are the histology appendices to the toxicity study"). Worse, clinical and commercial hegemony would prevail, with abrupt changes in clinical trials or trade dress, coinciding with changes of individual project team membership. Most of the people present could not make a useful contribution for most of the time compounded by the fact that project team meetings would be arranged by calendar, even if there was nothing new to talk about, rather than by following the milestones and decision points in the project. It gets worse: the submission of the registration dossier was seen as the conclusion of the project task with little attention to the need to have an active project team to answer regulatory questions, let alone support marketing, launch, and life cycle management. These war stories, which we all share, are very instructive in hindsight because by not repeating these errors, a coherent way of working can be devised.

So, where to start? Before assembling a project team, the first task is to define the target profile.

IMPORTANCE OF THE TARGET PROFILE

A significant change in pharma came about when the deficiencies of the linear model (candidate molecule transmutes into new product) became apparent with products being registered, which the companies' marketing divisions just did not want to promote. No effort had been made to establish a vision of success to which the scientific and commercial arms of the business could both subscribe. The target profile is an important tool in achieving this vision and the emphasis is now to plan back from where the organization sees itself at a point in the future. It does not guarantee success but it helps augment value, reduce risk, and mitigate against failure.

The first requirement for any project team, then, is to establish a target profile. For the organization at large, it is the basis for establishing the position within the portfolio of projects and becomes the vehicle to attract senior sponsorship and to focus the attention of all the stakeholders. It provides legitimacy for the project at the highest level and ensures that work is knowingly undertaken in its name. At the operational level, it provides a concrete target for the efforts of the project team and, with it, purpose is established. Target profiles are dealt with elsewhere in this book (refer chap. 2) but let us remind ourselves that it has both commercial and scientific elements—the commercial elements relate to intellectual property, market projections, cost of goods and margin, measures of value (net present value (NPV), return on investment (ROI), etc.) and so on and the scientific aspects relate to the mode of action, dose, frequency, route of administration, measures of efficacy, and safety and health outcomes. The target profile is thus a hybrid, with the extrinsic factors supporting the commercial case (and largely confidential to the company), while the intrinsic factors going to build the summary of product characteristics, which will exist in the public domain. The reason for reminding ourselves of these basic features is that the project team is dealing simultaneously with both public, and company-confidential information and the team must understand these differences when communicating about the product under development with the wider audience. It also highlights another dilemma for the project team: the need to plan for success while knowing that intrinsic properties of the molecule, hitherto unrevealed, can bring a project to an abrupt halt at any time. Project teams should also seek to "fail fast"—perform those tasks likely to give maximum information at minimum cost about the future viability of the project.

Finally, another advantage of a target profile is that it helps decide what should or should not be undertaken in the name of the project. There is always a tendency for what the military calls "mission creep," which refers to the accretion of additional tasks to the project, small but significant changes to the overall objective and so on. By maintaining the target profile, it helps distinguish between what should be undertaken in the name of the project and what should not be. It may still be undertaken but that is a functional responsibility and is not the responsibility of the project.

THE PROJECT MANAGER

In pharma, it is unusual for a project manager to appear out of thin air. Normally, they emerge from the organization as functional experts who have demonstrated some natural flair for working in cross-functional teams and especially project subteams (discussed later), which often act as good incubators for potential project managers. Much has been written about project managers and it is not part of this discussion to dwell on the role but suffice it to say that they need a whole battery of skills, most of which look dangerously like oxymorons:

- *Understands strategic drug development, yet appreciative of the detailed work of the functional experts.*
- *Commands the respect and unequivocal support of the senior management sponsors but equally approachable to the most junior stakeholders of the project.*
- *Politically astute but avoids politicizing the project.*
- *Understands what are the risks but not overly conservative in approach.*
- *Thinks globally but acts locally.*
- *Leverages the individual talents of the functional experts, whatever the national or cultural background, to the benefit of the project by agreeing objectives and setting individual expectations but at the same time encourages team cohesion and mutual support and respect.*
- *Champions the project but knows when to stop.*
- *Absorbs data but communicates knowledge.*

The list goes on. One significant failing of project manager training has been the undue emphasis on process management. In truth, essential though they are, bar charts, risk registers, and financial spreadsheets do not make for project management in themselves; it has got far more to do with the soft side of managing people and there is no doubt that the most successful project managers have an uncanny knack of drawing people to them and persuading them to devote their efforts to the common purpose. Functional experts, with purpose declared, know what needs to be done but it is the linking across the functional groups where the project manager should spend the majority of their time: *"Manage the interfaces. . . and the experts will look after themselves."* It also follows that project managers, whatever their scientific prowess, must not become personally involved in the project science but must work through the project experts. It can be frustrating but if a project manager becomes personally embroiled, then it is certain that this will be at the expense of overall control of the project. It is unlikely that such a job can be sustained except at a relatively senior level of the organization but that does not prevent some organizations from attempting to manage projects at a more junior level: the task then is not project management but some form of low-level project coordination with functional hegemony and all the problems that entails. Sponsors need to be clear about what their expectations of the project manager are and appoint accordingly. Equally, project managers mature into their roles and the authority they command develops over time as people at all levels experience just how the project is managed.

Perhaps one way to make sense of the project manager's role is to redefine the role to that of knowledge manager (3). It is beyond the scope of this chapter to progress too far down this route but thinking of a project as a complex system directed to acquiring and communicating knowledge goes a long way to underpin that elusive rationale for project team working. Projects are nothing if they are not generators of knowledge.

MATRIX WORKING

Projects draw on wide-ranging expertise and it is not practicable to group all the skills required in a single functional department or even in a company. Large pharma companies may have all the resource required internally but then it only becomes integrated at the highest level and it is just not possible for the chief executive officer, for instance, to be the project manager (although some do behave that way!) and some fix has to be found to make the system work. Functional departments, especially in a large pharma, usually find competition from several different projects for their limited resources and this was how two-dimensional matrix representation emerged. By having a representative on each active project, the functional department could make better estimates of when and how much resource would be required for each project and make some sense of the need to budget and schedule tasks. This, however, puts real responsibility with the project representative (who might have to turn out for several projects if resources are limited). Historically, much of the impetus for matrix working came from the U.S. Military in the 1960s when the then Secretary of State for Defense insisted that there be a point contact for the negotiation of military contracts rather than being pushed around from expert to expert or company to company, according to the particular aspect of the contract under discussion. However, the fact remains that there is a fundamental conflict in the way we organize for product development. Even companies that set out to work with cross-functional teams as the organizational model, eventually fall back to functional hierarchy as the organization gets bigger and matrix working can all too often become a conceit. Every one pays lip service to cross-functional working and to the autonomy of the project team but, in reality, project teams have no autonomy whatsoever and it is the functional management that calls the shots. However, things are changing again and we will revisit this topic towards the end of this chapter.

PROJECT TEAM MEMBERSHIP

Another significant departure from textbook descriptions of teams is project team membership. It is not common for a project manager to hand pick a development team; they may have some idea about whom they would like or not like on their team, based on experience, but usually the functional manager has little choice from which to make an appointment. Additionally, functional expertise (the reason for appointment to a project team) is not automatically associated with good team skills. Another scenario is that a project manager may have to be changed, in which case the incoming project manager inherits an established team and has to find a way to work with it. Even popular methods such as Belbin or Myers-Briggs come unstuck because while they can be instructive to understand the range of team types and the individual personalities you have inherited, it does not make much sense to decide whether you want a chemist who is a "coordinator" or a regulatory affairs professional who is a "monitor evaluator" and so on—you would probably want them to be there for what they are—specialists. Therefore, project managers rarely appoint their teams and do not "control" them in a hierarchical management sense. Representatives will vary in seniority, in experience, and in style and temperament. Add to this the growing need to manage project teams in alliances between companies, clinical research organizations (CROs), and other organizations and the potential difficulties for traditional team models compound exponentially. However, there is a very positive way forward and that is for the project manager to encourage empowerment of the individual, promote situational leadership, and understand how team types work together (then Belbin and Myers-Briggs, for instance, do come into their own). It means that for each component of the project, the expert assumes leadership. When talking regarding toxicology, the toxicology representative holds the floor and leads the team because that is what they are there to do and no one else can do it. As one senior manager once said to me (paraphrased)—"They may be a load of awkward individuals, but they're the only awkward individuals you've got, so get on with it." In fact, a key attribute of a great project manager is the ability to do constructive business with all the stakeholders he/she comes to face within the project system and ensure that they in turn are able to network across the team to the overall benefit of the project.

So, for a rapid, flexible response, project teams and subteams should have

- inclusive membership,
- flexible membership evolving by stage of development,
- membership determined by the tasks to be done, and
- meetings frequency and agenda determined by the tasks.

In addition, subteams should form and dissolve rapidly according to the task at hand—because teams have no purpose unless they have a purpose! Having spelt out the difficulties of forming the "ideal" core project team, there is no reason why one cannot describe the ideal profile of a project representative, which might look something like this:

Expertise:	*Characteristics:*
Functional	Proactivity
Technical	Commitment/ownership
Drug development	Objectivity
	Forward thinking
Skills:	Credibility/trust
Communication skills	Good judgment
Decision making	Self confidence
Problem solving	Team Player
Lateral thinking	Resilient to change
Organizational skills	Sense of humor
Negotiating/influencing skills	Ability to challenge

PROJECT HIERARCHY

Another improvement in cross-functional team working has been to distinguish between the strategic, the operational, and the functional level within the project. It is highly confusing if all aspects of the project are discussed in the same mêlée. The strategic intent is agreed at the portfolio level, the operational ("block diagram") content is discussed at project level, and the functional content is delivered by the expert subteams. This hierarchy is a very useful aid to project management: as mentioned earlier, but worth repeating, it saves the team getting embroiled in strategic discussions at one extreme ("I don't know why we are doing this project...") and detailed discussion at the other ("Here are the comprehensive histopathology results from that unremarkable 28-day oral toxicology study in the rat we have just completed...").

EVOLUTION OF SUBTEAM WORKING

As the matrix view emerged, it became obvious that much practical work on a particular project could be managed in a functional area without the need to involve the project team at large. Thus, because the planning hierarchy allows a clear separation of the strategic, operational, and functional aspects of the project, it also leads to a more coherent model for project team evolution. However, this was not the end of the story because the project was still being driven forward on the basis of "we have started so we will continue."

NETWORKED SUBTEAMS

A good outward sign of a mature project team is the existence of a wide range of networked subteams that form and dissolve according to the task at hand. It is just not possible to use a command structure for project team working where everything is controlled centrally. The clinical supplies team, for instance, will have membership drawn from chemistry, manufacturing, and controls, and clinical research: it is formed to deal with specific issues concerning clinical supplies and does not require the routine attendance of the nonclinical safety expert or the marketing representative or even the project manager—although he/she should be aware of its existence and should be in the communication loop over its deliberations. The team has a defined purpose and, within the overall remit of the project, will organize its own activities accordingly. Such teams are not the same as functional subteams (CMC, nonclinical, etc.) and are themselves cross-functional matrix teams but they exist at the functional and not the operational level.

FURTHER EVOLUTION OF THE PROJECT TEAM

A constant question is the extent to which project teams are empowered. Within the project, authority and power derive from the purpose for which it was established and the knowledge of the project team members. However, different organizations allow project teams to have different degrees of latitude, usually through budgetary control, and they range from the fully autonomous "tiger team" through to the team under direct functional control. Most mainstream pharma teams hover somewhere in the lightweight to heavyweight area (4) but rarely hold their own budgets. In fact, in an inversion of the "Responsible, Accountable, Consult, Inform (RACI)" model, project managers can be held accountable for the work but have no control— managerial or budgetary—over those responsible for doing the work!

PRACTICAL ASPECTS OF MANAGING THE PROJECT TEAM

No project team is alike and "best practice" is likely to be a chimera because it is so intimately bound up with people and circumstances at a point in time. Recognizing and understanding this complexity does, however, give good guidance to the project manager on how to work effectively. But late in the day and despite the significant advances in project team organization, such is pharma development that the candidate molecule may yet reveal properties that mean it cannot be transmuted into a successful product.

THE DISTRIBUTED PROJECT TEAM IS THE NORM

Many textbook descriptions of successful teams rely on colocation. This is just not the case with pharma project teams. With widespread consolidation and outsourcing, it is common to find functional units geographically scattered and with little or no vertical integration of all the resources required within one geographical location.

One systematic description of the space between individuals describes the range from intimate (<0.5 m) through personal, social, and then public with the colocated team members being no more than 15 m apart (5). Distances larger than this (different floors in the same building, different buildings) define a distributed team and different sites, cities, countries, and even continents produce much the same difficulties. Because of the way pharma has evolved, different expert groups are physically separated for any number of reasons and the competent team will find that communication needs are similar (laying aside cultural aspects for the time being) whether talking on the phone to someone at another floor of your building or half way across the world. A staircase can be as significant a barrier as an international air flight. It is a waste of time seeking a holy grail of "colocated team behaviors" when the distributed team is the norm. (2)

EFFECTIVE WORKING IN TEAMS

We have already concluded that pharma project teams are teams dispersed by time, geography, and culture; so, how do we encourage them to work effectively? A reminder now that the project team gains its authority from the purpose for which it was established, its power from the knowledge that it has to complete the task and from the reason for which it was established. Having said that, we now find that some very traditional practices become crucial to successful operations.

Firstly, do not forget the hierarchy within the project. Contribute to strategy setting by all means, but the project's existence has been established at the portfolio level and remains legitimate until told otherwise. Certainly, the team can help shape a strategic decision as new information emerges but do not waste valuable time contemplating your own existence. At the other extreme, do not get embroiled in the fine detail of the expert work when the core project team cannot make a useful contribution. Do not expect the pharmacists to make a contribution to the derivation of the data management and statistical analysis plan for phase 3. However, at the operational level where the core project team should operate, overall integration of the plans for secondary manufacture has to be fully integrated with the need to supply clinical trials supplies and this is where the core team can make the significant contribution by integrating the development operation.

Secondly, be clear about who does what. This is where the RACI approach is so useful. For every task, list out who is responsible for actually doing the work (the functional expert), who is accountable for ensuring the work is done (the functional manager), then who needs to be consulted (stakeholders involved in some way with either commissioning the work or reliant on it being completed and who could hold a legitimate veto), and who needs to be informed (those who will not veto the work but will be impacted in some way). Not considered in the conventional RACI analysis is another important group—those who are not involved and whose opinion is not sought. The matrix is full of people with opinions about what and how things should or should not be done and it is sensible to be clear whose opinion to heed and whom, politely, to ignore.

TEAM DECISION MAKING

Far too much time can be lost in debating matters just not relevant to the current stage of the project. There are plenty of texts which describe methods for reaching consensus in teams but suffice it to say that there are matters that are already agreed, usually at a strategic level ("We are working on this project because. . ."), and there are matters where the decision is not required at this time ("We will take a decision in six months time when the results are available. . ."). It then leaves the team free to concentrate on matters where a decision has to be reached in the immediate future ("Based on the results of the milestone toxicology study, the project team recommends that we progress to first time in humans. . .").

Time wasted in unnecessary attention to detail also occurs if there is inappropriate precision in the project schedules. Software products can famously predict what will happen to the minute on a date several years into the future but such is the nature of the planning horizon that this is not realistic. A sensible project decision about future dates will be mindful of the appropriate precision with more generous limits some time out (5 years $\pm$ 1 quarter) that are hardened up as milestones draw closer (6 months $\pm$ 2 weeks) and so on.

EXTERNAL PARTNERS AND ALLIANCE MANAGEMENT (PROJECT MANAGEMENT WRIT LARGE)

There is a view that project managers are born and not bred and one hallmark of the consummate project manager is that they like people. In case of distributed project teams, with sponsors and stakeholders from other companies (both project team and functional management), it is just as essential, as with in-house teams, to know them as individuals, to know how they "sit" in the organization's hierarchy, and to gauge their level of interest in the work you are doing. It may take time to discern but it is time well spent. An appreciation of national and/or cultural differences is also essential. It can help mitigate stress when, for instance, there is a standoff between a team member who, typical for his or her nation, expects an immediate response to a question posed in a team meeting and the responder who comes from a nation where the culture is to reflect with colleagues on a question and not answer immediately. Recognizing that such deep-seated differences cannot be resolved immediately allows rapid conflict resolution because the sensitive project manager can see the situation arising, understand the basis, and defuse. With the rapid rise in so-called alliance management, there are also differences to the more established model of the procurer or provider that exists in relationships with contract research organizations (conventionally managed by functional specialists). In alliance management, where there may be a strategic partnership between two or more organizations of equals, the "cultural" sensitivity extends to an appreciation of "how things are done here" and the knowledge that the room for maneuver for a project team member may be very different in another company.

It is just not sensible to overlook such differences and the project manager must find ways to work with it and not against it.

As with all team evolution, alliances will experience the "forming, storming, norming, performing, and finally adjourning" ritual. In such circumstances, the project manager will be sensitive to what the alliance will tolerate in the form of documentation. Project status reports, for instance, may start off as quite simple expressions of intent and, as the alliance matures, can then proceed to more sophisticated documents as members become comfortable with the joint working practices.

MEETINGS, MEETINGS, MEETINGS...

If there was ever an occasion where a traditional meetings procedure is required, it is the pharma project team meeting.

What We Do but Should Not

We are all used to winging it—a chance meeting of some individuals at the coffee point, some of whom may be in the project core (operational) team, a flip-chart, an ad hoc agenda, covering for absent colleagues because we "know where they are coming from" and Hey Presto! a decision, which may or may not be communicated elsewhere. Let us not deny it, this is very easy to fall into and we all do it but it is just not good enough for the distributed project core team.

Setting the Agenda

We all know how tedious the unending stream of meetings is but we must like them because we always turn up! However, some simple attention to detail can make the whole experience more acceptable. The first question to ask is: why is the meeting required? Then, what level of detail needs to be considered? Is this an expert functional group meeting or a town hall general briefing on the state of the project? Who needs to attend and are they available? Has the agenda been circulated in a timely fashion so that those attending can consult within their expert groups? Have the communications been set up and advised? Face-to-face, teleconference, Web meeting, videoconference? Time zones? Languages? Translator? Would a facilitator be of assistance to the project manager? Timekeeper? Scribe? Action points or a verbatim account?

When to Hold a Meeting?

Meetings, like death, never occur at convenient times. Things have happened and information is available but other things are in the process of being done and other things are planned for the future and nothing has yet happened. So, the time is never convenient but, as a rule of thumb, link meetings to the natural history of the project—at milestones and decision points and when the team may have to report into higher management.

The Meeting Itself

Here, the project manager will stretch his/her people skills to the full: by encouraging situational leadership, the project manager can hopefully elicit a full contribution from each member present, in spite of the fact that they come in all shapes and sizes ("subordinate maturity"). Each functional expert enjoys uninterrupted sovereignty for their contribution but remember that representatives vary in their level of empowerment and it is wise to be mindful of the level of commitment that a representative can sustain. If the representative is Vice President (VP) toxicology, then if they say the toxicology can start at a certain time and be completed within a given period, that is probably going to be a recordable action but do not bounce a representative who does not bring that authority into agreeing decision, which will be immediately undone when they return and report into their departmental managers. That is why timely circulation of the agenda is so important: a functional representative can shape the decision and come prepared. Always record actions in a decision log and agree with team members regarding how much time they need to report back into their functional areas to get ratification.

Action points should be circulated as rapidly as possible and the project manager should up not only the decision log but also the risk register. The project manager should also drive the actions in a timely manner

So, keep the meetings small and issue-based, leverage the full network of team members in order to develop the cross-functional view, gain a clear definition of accountabilities (RACI—discussed earlier) and feel enabled to expand the network to address specific agenda-driven requirements. Have an efficient mechanism for communication of information between the core team and the subteams. In terms of human behavior, effective communication has an unexpected beneficial side effect: no longer will team and subteam meetings be overattended with multiple representatives from a single function. Often, the reason for overattendance is that functional experts feel it is the only way to gain information about what is going on in a project. Once all stakeholders have a common understanding of what is going on, the clamor to attend meetings "for information" falls away as the functional members gain the confidence that others are contributing what is required and can be left to get on with that which they know best.

At the End of the Meeting

Take the time to conduct a brief review of how the meeting went. Without interruption or comment allow all present to contribute comments on what they thought went well and what they would do differently next time (a less confrontational way of describing what went badly!). Such a review itself contributes to team building and allows all to reflect on how to do things better next time around.

Communicating Decisions

Following a meeting, there is the need to communicate. Project managers need to overcommunicate rather than undercommunicate and they should be acutely aware of the people with whom they need to communicate. It is not just the project team itself but also sponsors and stakeholders often at a senior level in the organization. The project manager must network tirelessly at all levels of the organization in order to maintain active interest and support for the project. There is a downside of course and the project manager must strive for objectivity. The project manager must champion the project but at the same time (another oxymoron) be sensitive to new information that may affect the position of the project within the company's portfolio and, if harsh decisions need to be made, be prepared to shape them for the sponsors and stakeholders even if the recommendation is that the project should cease.

Finally, it is worth reflecting that there are three types of general communication in which a project manager indulges:

- Coordination of tasks and transfer of the emergent technical information
- Motivating the team and inspiring management support
- Building the body of project knowledge by consultation and by teaching

PROJECT START-UP

We should not forget that a special case of the project team meeting is the project start-up. All of the techniques for running effective team meetings described above need to be deployed but there is the additional requirement that the new team needs to knit together and start working effectively as soon as possible. Ideally, start-ups should be held face-to-face and with the assistance of a competent facilitator. With international teams and distributed membership, there are significant cost barriers to face-to-face meetings but so crucial is the start-up that every effort should be made to secure funding to allow it to happen. Practical experience reveals time and time again that an effective face-to-face start-up meeting with time for the group to socialize outside of the formal business pays dividends over and over again for the continuing conduct of the project business. Once these human relationships are established, it makes distance working and the use of teleconferencing or videoconferencing that much easier. There will be the traditional team behaviors of "forming, storming, norming, and performing." These should not be overlooked and the project manager should be sensitive to the dynamics. In pharma project teams, there is often some mitigation of these effects because many project team members will have already served on other teams and are already used to working in a cross-functional environment. With experience, project members acquire "transferable team skills" and are able to deploy these in new situations. This can be leveraged by the project manager and, with their assistance, can be used to assimilate new team members who have less experience in cross-functional working.

Distance Working for Teams—What Medium?

With the advances in communications technology, videoconferencing has become a much more reliable and affordable way to communicate but is it actually the best way? Experienced project managers will tell you that for a mature team teleconferencing has much to commend it because there is less distraction from the body language of videoconference participants not actually engaged in a particular conversation. The audio route allows for more concentration and focus and the video channel can be replaced with more useful desk-to-desk conferencing technologies such as shared working space for document review or electronic white boarding.

ENGAGING WITH FUNCTIONAL MANAGERS

The relationship between the project manager and the functional manager is one of the most important and probably one of the most fraught within the matrix system. The reason for this is described in the introduction to this chapter and many of the day-to-day problems actually derive from the issue of control. The traditional view of control is that the hierarchical manager can order a particular outcome but we know this is just not possible to guarantee. No amount of cajoling will result in the discovery of a "clean" toxicology profile when the result is dependant upon the hitherto unrevealed properties of the candidate drug. The role of the functional manager is actually the reverse of deterministic control: it is to manage uncertainty. While a functional manager can plot a critical path for their expert activities, it is usually the case that perturbations to the critical path come from areas outside of the influence of the expert group. There may be a terrific timetable for conducting the clinical trial but if the clinical trials supplies are delayed by a failure in actives manufacture, there is nothing the clinical functional leader can do about it. A very popular topic is risk identification and contingency planning but there are limits to how much this can be built into the development plan because so many of the tasks are "new," without precedent (except in the general sense) and are capable of tripping you up. Furthermore, popular response to the need for contingency plans—dual sourcing—can be extremely expensive, for example, for the manufacture of active substance and, in truth, although we all play lip service to it, the opportunities are not that common and so a number of pharma development activities (including actives manufacture) have to be considered as "at risk" investment.

So, what is the nature of the relationship between the project manager and the functional manager? It all lies in the empowerment of the project represen-tative to deliver the task to time, to cost, and to quality (i.e., meeting the target profile). The functional manager provides the resources, physical and financial to their staff, within an environment to maximize the chances of success. Over and above this, the functional manager provides the working environment with all the necessary facilities along with the essential support for the individual in the form of personal management, coaching, training, and development. This becomes even more sophisticated when strategic planning is used to decide what studies should be done and in what order so that maximum information needed to progress development is collected without entailing unnecessary expenditure. Thus, it makes sense not to engage in long term carcinogenicity studies before a phase 1/2 proof-of-concept study has been undertaken but other choices are more subtle; precisely what toxicology package is required to support phase 1 will be compound and indication-specific and this is where the expertise of the functional manager will be called upon because it is not within the remit of the project manager to give such an advice.

So, the functional manager allocates resources to the project and advises on costs and also ensures scientific robustness, timeliness, and quality of product development. They collaborate with the project manager in issues resolution and conflict management. They ensure that the functional (subteam) matrix is operating successfully.

A Word About Stretch Targets

We all want the projects to deliver on time, on cost, and to target profile and there is also pressure from management to perform even more quickly. Stretch targets, however, are a dangerous threat. Any estimate of time has a risk associated with it and is dependant partly on history ("We have done this before. . .") and partly on the expertise applied to a new situation ("It is likely to be different because of these factors. . ."). There is always a risk that a time target will not be met and time and money will be used to correct it. To apply a stretch target is therefore to increase the risk that the target will not be met. It is wholly wrong for senior management to set one-sided stretch targets without the implicit acceptance that if something does go wrong, it will go wrong big time. This is not to say that project teams should be given unending durations for tasks but to recognize that all undertakings have a risk. This is one argument for using the critical chain methods for project planning, which says that rather than each expert function adding on their own contingency padding, the organization recognizes that not all this contingency is required and pools its risks, to be taken up by whatever function runs into trouble. This requires understanding of the problem by senior management and it has been argued that if senior managers really did understand the nature of risk and contingency planning, then the same result could be obtained with more conventional critical path techniques.

RESOLVING TEAM CONFLICT

As in all walks of life, conflict can arise in project teams and there are any number of techniques that might be applied to achieve resolution. However, when looked at objectively, it is apparent that conflict in project teams usually arises from one of two causes. Firstly, there are straightforward personality clashes between individual project managers, team members, sponsors, and stakeholders. In such cases, there is no alternative than that the individuals involved should sort out their differences and find a way to work together and, if they cannot, they need to be separated, usually be a redefinition of roles and responsibilities. My personal experience is that this is not that common and that the consummate project manager can spot the body language early on and take appropriate action. Far more common is the conflict that arises because the task has not been adequately defined and there is a mismatch of expectations: the project and the expert function, for instance, may have a very different view about the anticipated output of a particular task. In these circumstances, the simplest remedy is for all parties to remind themselves what it is they are committed to and assure alignment. Rather than being the point of conflict, the project representative then becomes the focal point for project manager and functional manager to agree on the correct course of action and it is not acceptable to just leave the representative to try and sort out the differences unaided. A bigger problem occurs when there is a failure of alignment in the functional hierarchy. Project expert and immediate line management may agree upon a course of action but that is not consolidated at higher levels and the conflict only surfaces when a functional expert who is also a project sponsor takes umbrage at the direction a project is taking when it comes up for sponsor review at, say, a portfolio review meeting. This is a failure of management and should be dealt with by the chief executive—it is not something that the project manager can resolve unaided. If there is a genuine difference in perception then the target profile becomes an essential tool to resolution, with the assistance of senior sponsors of the project as appropriate.

REWARD AND RECOGNITION

The greatest trap that senior managers can fall into is to single out the project manager for special reward when a project is successful—at intermediate milestones as well as at completion. It overlooks the basic fact that successful project managers get there be leveraging the considerable efforts of all project team members and, if true to type, the project manager will be acutely embarrassed by singular attention. Certainly, team members should be rewarded for their expert efforts through conventional line function mechanisms—pay rise, bonus, promotion, or whatever mechanism is available (and this will also apply to the manager) but conspicuous project reward should be for the team as a whole and can take place in many ways; often a team celebration (special dinner, company reception, etc.) is all that is needed. And what is more, the vexed question of who should and should not attend is invariably solved—the team itself. Function representatives can usually be relied on to identify who from their subteams should represent the function in any celebration.

What is not so obvious is reward for failure. A project may not be successful but correct and timely decision-making to terminate activities that would otherwise continue to sap company resources is also worthy of reward and should be treated as such.

Poor performance at the project expert level needs to be addressed and the project manager needs to maintain ongoing contact with the functional managers so that any deficiencies are apparent early on. However, this is not necessarily such an easy issue to discern. Project experts themselves are reliant on their own subteams for delivering the project task and there may be systematic problems for which the functional expert cannot be held personally responsible and the truth is that many more project "failings" have diffuse causes and are not rightly attributed to individual culpability. This is not an excuse for adopting a Panglossian view of project endeavor and there will be occasional incidences of unacceptable performance but it is too easy to punish the innocent on such occasions and this should not be tolerated.

PROJECT TEAM MATURITY

A common fallacy into which we must not fall is that project teams mature with time and perform at ever-increasing levels of effectiveness. The goal is for the "high-performing team" and the team members develop skills that can be passed to other teams to the overall benefit of the organization at large. But this does not always happen: effective teams require continuous maintenance and if the project manager fails to supply the necessary momentum, the team will fall back into its "functional silo" mode, to the detriment of the project. The dangers are everywhere, especially during mergers and acquisitions. The dangers include

- a sudden change in sponsor, with failure to restate the legitimacy of the project,
- an abrupt handover of responsibility to a new project manager, and
- ad hoc changes to core project team membership.

All of these factors can seriously destabilize an effective project team. It may well be that the legitimacy of the project will be brought into question during a portfolio review and that the project will close. But if the project is to continue, senior management must take great care to ensure that such changes do not weaken the effectiveness of the project team and should devote special attention to stabilizing the efforts of the project manager and the project team.

WHAT OF THE FUTURE?

Despite my observation that matrix working is an artificial construct applied to hierarchical organizations to enable cross-functional working, there are now strong signs that a new reality is dawning. As companies have sought to delayer management structures in the quest for efficiency and cost containment, management structures are becoming lower, flatter, and populated with self-directed professionals. These professionals are engaged in exchanging knowledge. Knowledge working is the way forward but it is a subject in its infancy. Whether by intent or not, these organizations can only function effectively by extensive cross-functional networking and this means the structures within which project management can flourish to the benefit of the organization are becoming the only structures with which to contend (6). A theoretical rationale for this phenomenon is now being supplied by study of the behavior of so-called complex adaptive systems. Perhaps the greatest failure of traditional management has been to expect linear predictability of behavior in the systems they manage. This is possible but not certain with repetitive processes; however, it is not the case with product development where we are "hostages to the properties of the compound." The systems are innately complex, bordering on the chaotic, and new ways to deal with this are long overdue (3). While one has to be careful not to overinterpret the superficial similarities with chemical and biological evolution, there is much to be gained by looking at the phenomenon of self-organization in human society, which reaches a high level within effective project teams. Intuitive project managers have always known it. They were born with it.

An Example of a Project Team Charter

It is assumed that the company is committed to developing its assets through the deployment of product development project teams—these are engines of the business.

A core project team is established whenever there is a need to deliver a specific objective that draws upon expertise from a variety of different functions not under direct common line management and where team members can often be separated by time, geography, or culture.

For a product development project team, the requirement is to devise and execute a plan to achieve optimal development and maximize the commercial value of the asset (medicine and/or delivery device) for the company—delivering the new product to the agreed time, cost, and target profile.

Legitimacy of project teams

Project teams derive their authority from the purpose for which they were established and their power from the knowledge that the team representatives possess.

Depending on the stage of development, projects report into either a Center for Excellence in Drug Discovery (candidate selection through to proof of concept) or a Therapeutic Area Strategy Team (proof of concept through to life cycle management).

Principles

The principles of core project team operation are observed in the product development process and are as follows:

Purpose—achieving the target profile by undertaking interdependent tasks
 designed to produce concrete evidence about the asset
People—independent team representatives from the functions, taking responsibility in the team for their expertise and often drawn across different
 levels of seniority in the organization
Links—communicating across interfaces using multiple media and sustained
 by mutual trust

It is unlikely that a core project team will have more than 8 to15 members
since the bulk of the operational work will be conducted by project subteams
but membership is inclusive rather than exclusive and is guided by the task at
hand.

The principles apply widely and can be variously applied to early stage
development (e.g., program teams) as well as project subteams (e.g., chemistry,
manufacturing and controls (CMC)) and other cross-functional groups outside
of product development (IT project teams, etc.).

Project team purpose

Define the target profile or, if this has already been established, ensure understanding of the target profile and how it links forward into the intended
 summary of product characteristics.
Prepare a product development strategy and recommend it to the sponsors for
 approval.
Plan development activities and timelines, establish the resource and budgetary
 requirements, and achieve consensus based on the expert view so that
 the functional areas share a commitment to undertake and deliver the
 work.
Undertake risk analysis and, by priority, prepare contingency plans for potential
 outcomes to future project activities.
Define options and make specific recommendations on changes to agreed plans
 for approval by senior matrix management.
Keep development process on time and within budget.
Monitor the emerging asset profile against the target product profile.
Ensure timely and effective product launches.
Ensure efficient and effective life cycle management of the asset.
Communicate project status to management, advise management of project
 requirements, and implement decisions approved by senior matrix man-
 agement.

Project team people

Project teams draw on the expertise of the functions to advance the team
purpose. Team members

commit to the project team and accept accountability for team deliverables.

represent their function by actively participating in core team and subteam meetings and assuming situational leadership when discussing issues for which they are recognized as the expert.

understand commercial goals and impact of department activities on the target product profile.

provide functional plans to agreed timelines.

track the progress of functional activities informing the team of any possible deviation from agreed strategy and timings.

accept and resolve action items in a timely manner as agreed to at project team meetings.

ensure that all advice given to the project team is supported at the highest appropriate level within the function and, if there is disagreement, engage the functional manager and the project manager in the constructive resolution of the issue.

demonstrate a sense of urgency regarding communication of headline data, emerging issues, and competitive information.

make effective presentations to project team, management committees, and external customers, as required.

Project team links

The project team is at the center of an extensive network of functions and individuals requiring access to project information. Not all those in the extended network are required to participate in decision making. Decision making in project teams or subteams is effective when

the right people are present,
the information is shared with a common understanding, and
the timing and business objective for the decision are aligned.

Project managers and team representatives should convene both regular, focused core team meetings for decision making and, whenever needed, larger meetings aimed at information sharing. Attendance at a meeting will be driven by the objective and the agenda content.

The project manager

Accountabilities

Delivery of the project to time, cost, and target profile.

Responsibilities

Provide leadership of transnational project teams.

Manage the optimal development of multiple projects from candidate selection through to successful product launches and full life cycle management.

Ensure effective forecasting and tracking of project resources.

For the specific project to be lead, build commitment of the project team to the target profile and lead the team in setting and continuously reviewing the emergent asset profile against the target product profile, the development strategy, budget, and time lines.

Ensure team expertise is fully available and utilized.

Develop the talent of team members to work in projects.

Encourage and empower situational leadership and delegate specific project-related activities and responsibilities to the project manager, project team subgroup, and/or project team representatives.

Seek to empower project team representatives while appreciating variation in seniority, experience, style, and temperament.

Critically monitor project progress against milestones and decision points. Proactively and continuously evaluate the project for risks and prepare contingency plans for anticipated outcomes. Manage deviations and exceptions and regularly interrogate ways of accelerating development.

Present to senior R&D and corporate management committees project proposals/plans/updates and issues and recommendations and communicate decisions to the project team.

Provide supervision of the project support office in the planning and coordination of projects.

The project support office

Responsibilities

Work with project manager and the team to develop an integrated development plan.

Provide comprehensive planning and tracking support for project manager and project team(s).

Assure implementation of standard project management and financial systems and processes.

Work with the project manager and the team to diagnose potential risks to the development and prepare contingency plans. Actively track progress to determine whether contingency plans need to be initiated.

Ensure team-training needs on the company processes are met.

Serve as project team secretariat and prepare minutes and action lists for team meetings. Meeting reports should be prepared around specific and time-bound action items, which should be tracked to resolution.

Be responsible for integration of project support activities (drug supply forecasts, clinical trial supply requirements).

Liaise with new product supply teams to assure and support technology transfer activities.

The functional manager

Responsibilities with respect to project teams

Appoint an appropriate representative of the function to the project team in collaboration with the project manager.

Coach the representative and ensure that team responsibilities are agreed with the project manager and reflected in the individual's performance development plan.

Ensure the representative is fully informed about issues relating to the function and possible courses of action in preparation for project team meetings.

Ensure that agreed team strategies are supported and resourced by the discipline.

Focus on communicating with the representatives to exchange information with the team and seek to resolve with them any specific issues relating to the function in a constructive manner involving, if necessary, the project manager.

REFERENCES

1. Hansen MT, von Oetinger B. Introducing T-shaped managers: knowledge management's next generation. Harvard Bus Rev (March 2001): 107.
2. Lipnack J, Stamps J. Virtual Teams: People Working Across Boundaries and Technology. 2nd edn. John Wiley & Sons, New York. 2000.
3. Kurtz CF, Snowden DJ. The new dynamics of strategy: sense-making in a complex and complicated world. J IBM Systems 2003;42(No. 3):462–483.
4. Clark KB, Wheelwright S. Organizing and leading "heavyweight" development teams. Calif Manage Rev 1992;34 (Suppl 3):9–28.
5. Allen T. Managing the Flow of Technology. Cambridge, MA: MIT Press, 1977, p. 47.
6. Bryan L, Joyce C. The 21st-century organization. The McKinsey Quarterly 2005; (No. 3):21–29.

9

Project Management and Outsourcing Drug Development

Jon Court
Fulcrum Pharma Developments Ltd., Hemel Hempstead, U.K.

Mark Fowler
Strategic Sourcing & Procurement, Amgen Inc, Thousand Oaks, California, U.S.A.

INTRODUCTION

Outsourcing is a business-critical process for most organizations irrespective of which business sector they operate in. There are good reasons for this since outsourcing can bring significant strategic and tactical benefits to businesses. The pharmaceutical sector is no exception to this rule and pharma companies, whatever their size, can achieve huge gains by adopting a well thought out outsourcing strategy. The global R&D outsourcing market is estimated to grow to $25 billion in 2007 (1) with continued double-digit growth project for the future. Needless to say, best-in-class project management of contracted drug development needs to be a core competency if the benefits of such a strategy are to be fully realized. This chapter focuses on project management and how it can be used to manage relationships with suppliers, reap the benefits, and deliver competitive advantage. The approach is generic, concentrates on optimizing the relationship between clients and vendors, and is broadly applicable to any outsourced development work.

Today, almost any aspect of drug development can be contracted out and the pharmaceutical industry continues to increase the amount of R&D that it outsources. All the large contract research and manufacturing organizations have shown growth over the last two years and the clinical research organizations have shown double-digit growth in 2004 and 2005 and this is set to continue (2). This trend is driving an improvement in business performance. The Tufts Centre for the Study of Drug Development analyzed contract research organization (CRO) usage by drug sponsors in 83 new drug applications submitted between 2000 and 2005. The study showed that extensive use of outsourced clinical research tended to result in projects being completed faster. They concluded, "clinical outsourcing offers a development speed advantage at comparable quality. And as the volume of clinical research activity continues to grow, CROs increasingly are providing a service that is essential to the long-term viability of the enterprise" (3,4).

For contracted development to be managed effectively the strategic objectives for going down the outsourcing route need to be understood. These could be one or more of the following (4):

- Lowering costs
- Improving business performance
- Accessing external expertise or skills
- Improving the quality and efficiency of the processes
- Achieving competitive advantage
- Creating new revenue sources

Understanding these objectives will influence the level and scope of project management and manager(s) required to deliver contracted development. While cost will almost always be an objective, understanding the noncost factors is at least as important. Small companies use contracting or outsourcing to facilitate growth as it saves on capital expenditure and allows management to concentrate on building the business and spread the risk inherent in building infrastructure before it is needed in full. Under these circumstances, "project management" will need to align itself with changing levels of internal staff, capabilities, and capacity throughout a project's life. Alternatively, large companies may use outsourcing to enable them to concentrate on their core business or access significant levels of resources and competency to improve efficiency, productivity, and, thus, overall competitiveness. Here the project management approach should take a broader view across several projects or processes. There are also other dimensions to consider. Suppliers and CROs come in all shapes and sizes and in fact the global CRO market remains highly fragmented with several thousand companies with revenues ranging from $1 million to $1 billion (2). Project managers need to understand the differing financial pressure that these suppliers are under (especially public companies) and structure contracts that benefit both parties. In such complex environments, project managers require specialized skill sets in order to succeed.

Experienced project managers who have used outsourcing effectively employ some simple pointers to maximize the benefits. While the relevance of these varies according to the size and maturity of an organization, they are worth considering and are as follows (5):

- Secure upfront agreement on expectations both for deliverables and in the manner and form of delivery (e.g., who does what, when, milestones, and critical time-points).
- Examine each stage of the value chain and focus on where there is a real scope for improvement, for example, cost, speed, and competence.
- Select the easiest and most urgent areas and examine the process in detail to determine how it can be done more effectively.
- Establish a short list of internal and external suppliers (the "supply chain"), map the process, systems, and personnel to be affected, and ensure common understanding across this matrix.

Underlying all of these considerations, project managers also need to understand the regulatory environment and the responsibilities of their employer as sponsors when conducting and managing outsourced drug development. The guidelines for this are documented and some of the constraints are summarized below:

- Within International Conference on Harmonization Good Clinical Practice (ICH GCP) Guidance—". . . the ultimate responsibility for the quality and integrity of the trial data always resides with the sponsor."
- In the EU under Directive 2005/28/EC—". . . the sponsor shall remain responsible for ensuring that the conduct of the trials and the final data generated by those trials comply with Directive 2001/20/EC as well as this Directive."
- The Organization of Economic Cooperative Development (OECD) Principles of Good Laboratory Practice (GLP) confirms "The sponsor must therefore assume an active role in confirming that all non-clinical health and environmental safety studies were conducted in compliance with GLP. Sponsors cannot rely solely on the assurances of test facilities they may have contracted to arrange or perform such studies."

OUTSOURCING STRATEGY

The level of project management skill, experience, and resources required for outsourcing will depend upon the type and scope of relationship you need with a supplier. Relationships may vary from tactical ad hoc, characterized as "as and when required" through to partnerships with mutual codependencies on each other (Fig. 1). The latter may be characterized by shared business goals such as both parties having an equity stake in a project or product or where there is sharing of infrastructure such as facilities. The level of relationship will depend upon the attitude of each party to risk and willingness to become dependent upon each other.

In simple terms, there are a number of ways to structure an outsourcing strategy and decision making; examples of these are shown below. This is not intended to be an exhaustive list but merely to illustrate some general relationships and strategies employed across organizations. As a general principle, organizations move through a staircase cascade with suppliers until an equilibrium is reached at a certain step on the cascade. Note though that any strategy may use a range of suppliers with whom the sponsoring company will likely have different

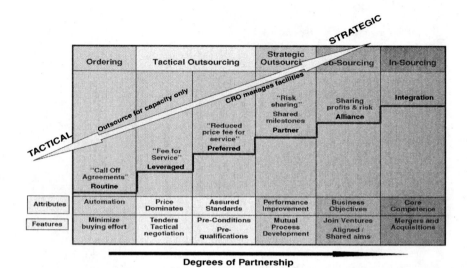

Degrees of Partnership

Figure 1 Outsourcing and range of deal structures. *Abbreviation*: CRO, contract research organization.

relationships and utilize different deal structures, some may be strategic and some tactical. The combination of these forms the outsourcing strategy.

To project manage a successful outsourcing strategy, whatever the deal structure, it is advisable to initially focus and prioritize high-expenditure category areas or bottleneck areas or functions critical to the project success. Examples of higher expenditure areas in clinical development will likely be clinical monitoring, data processing or management, and central laboratory while regulatory areas, report writing, or toxicology may be examples of critical bottleneck areas although not necessarily falling in the highest expenditure category.

In essence, the end result will be to balance and ensure clarity on commitments, sole source arrangements, and competitive tender while ensuring that an enabling infrastructure exists to support operational implementation of the strategy.

It is important that all project managers utilizing resources and services from external parties understand how supplier relationships are structured and managed. Too many relationships and constant flux in providers may well lead to confusion. For suppliers providing multiple services or goods, there may be value in appointing a specific relationship manager to "project manage" the relationship cross-functionally and monitor performance across projects while working with individual project managers.

RESOURCING FRAMEWORK FOR MANAGING OUTSOURCING

Resourcing frameworks need not be complex and, sometimes, simple competitive tender techniques "as and when required" may be perfectly sensible as shown in

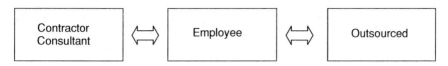

Figure 2   Resource pools.

Figure 1. For larger, complex, matrixed corporations and small biotech or pharma deploying a virtual strategy, a well-defined resourcing framework will allow clarity, focus, and the ability to flexibly resource across portfolio peaks and troughs in demand for capability and capacity. This is becoming ever more important as regulatory hurdles get higher and the demand to work in new geographic locations for reasons of cost and disease epidemiology increases. Further, companies, large and small, need to drive out capital efficiency while remaining nimble and responsive to changing economic conditions such as merger or acquisition and portfolio or product risk.

To be effective, a framework for taking resourcing decisions should be one that is well understood by all parties and adheres to the KISS principle—Keep It Simple Stupid. Sometimes, a clear and basic process done well can be more reliable and efficient than a fantastic but complex process that looks good on paper but is difficult to understand and operate in practice. The starting point for any resourcing framework is to first go back to basics and understand the baseline and define the desired outcome. Consider the world today within your organization and analyze the balance between the three main resource pools within the major functions that contribute to projects (Fig. 2).

The other key considerations for establishing a resourcing framework are as follows:

1. Decision making
   - How should resourcing decisions be taken across projects and within functions?
2. Economics
   - What are the fully loaded costs associated with each resource pool factoring in all fixed cost and variable overheads (e.g., labor, facility costs, management oversight, IT support, etc.)?
   - What should be the considerations for maximum and minimum desired fixed and variable cost, for example, employee headcount and infrastructure limitations?
3. Demand
   - What does the demand for services look like at least 12 months from now?
   - In which functions and geographies will likely capability and capacity be required?
   - What must be kept as part of the company's core competence to maintain its competitive position in the market in which it operates?

4. Supply chain efficiency and overhead
    *   How do functions connect up, do they deliver a streamlined sequence of events with minimal overhead?

Using outputs from these questions a framework can be crafted to facilitate effective resource management by taking a view on

*   employee levels by geography including any planned investments or divestments,
*   infrastructure available to support "on site" employees or contractors to enable optimal utilization of infrastructure investments,
*   consideration to workload balancing across multiple geographic facilities to optimize infrastructure usage of sunk fixed costs, and
*   coemployment risks around contractors and mitigation of these risks by setting maximum caps and conditions for contractor usage.

The following models (Fig. 3) illustrate four different resourcing frameworks for outsourcing in drug development. These models are followed by real examples that will provide an introduction to enabling infrastructure, relationship management, and governance, which will be covered in the remainder of the chapter.

Resourcing framework for outsourcing drug development Example 1.

Example 1: Functional Service Provider (No Internal Capacity)—Large Pharma and Central Laboratories

Over the past 10 years, many major pharma companies such as Pfizer, GSK, AstraZeneca, Roche, and Novartis have moved to a model of outsourcing all central laboratory services to specialist laboratories whose core business is central laboratory work. Significantly, this data can represent up to 70% of all data collected in clinical trials. The primary use of this data is to assess patient safety that represents a tremendous analytical and logistical challenge for both sponsors and central laboratories since it involves the transfer of data in specific formats to aggressive time lines and the highest possible quality standards.

In this scenario, central laboratory management focuses on the actual work of the sponsor with the laboratory rather than the selection. Depending on how well this cooperation is operationally managed and governed, the experience is that these partnership arrangements lead to a continuous process and thus service level improvement leading in turn to improved productivity and reduced costs.

To maintain market forces to drive the improvements mentioned, sponsors will typically maintain a partnership type arrangement with more than one but a minimal number of laboratories, the main reasons for this being the following:

*   To provide contingency and also meet scalability requirements from changing portfolio demand, i.e., to support effective capacity management
*   To access different laboratory strengths and capabilities such as technical experience in panels associated with specific therapeutic areas or operational experience in working in specific geographies

FSP = Functional Service Provider. Where single functions are outsourced across studies or programs to "best in class" functional expert suppliers. Can be local or offshore but permits sponsor's access to scalable competent resources who are trained and operate within sponsor's own systems and processes. This is usually operated as a staff augmentation model where resources reside and are managed within suppliers own infrastructure. FSP models are often referred to as commodity approaches as, in essence, functions are being commoditized and sourced and managed as such. Such models tend to require a high dependence on project management skills within sponsor as for any given project or study there may be a number of suppliers to be supply chain managed and output integrated.

Full Service = Where multiple functions are outsourced on a study or program basis to a single supplier. This is usually operated as a milestone deliverable model where supplier conducts the work to preagreed standards and payment is made for milestone deliverables. Such models require project management within the supplier but as all tasks remain within single supplier the overall project management complexity should be lower than with an FSP approach.

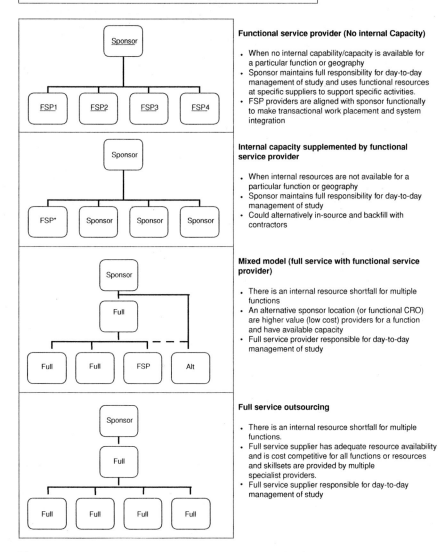

Functional service provider (No internal Capacity)

- When no internal capability/capacity is available for a particular function or geography
- Sponsor maintains full responsibility for day-to-day management of study and uses functional resources at specific suppliers to support specific activities.
- FSP providers are aligned with sponsor functionally to make transactional work placement and system integration

Internal capacity supplemented by functional service provider

- When internal resources are not available for a particular function or geography
- Sponsor maintains full responsibility for day-to-day management of study
- Could alternatively in-source and backfill with contractors

Mixed model (full service with functional service provider)

- There is an internal resource shortfall for multiple functions
- An alternative sponsor location (or functional CRO) are higher value (low cost) providers for a function and have available capacity
- Full service provider responsible for day-to-day management of study

Full service outsourcing

- There is an internal resource shortfall for multiple functions.
- Full service supplier has adequate resource availability and is cost competitive for all functions or resources and skillsets are provided by multiple specialist providers.
- Full service supplier responsible for day-to-day management of study

Figure 3   Resourcing frameworks for outsourcing drug development.

The number of laboratory partners required is usually driven by the capacity and capability requirements of the sponsor portfolio balanced against the upfront investment in setting up process for areas such as system platforms to support data transfer or management plus the operational overheads of managing the relationships and the associated issues or performance and governance with multiple organizations.

Resourcing framework for outsourcing drug development Example 2.

Example 2: Internal Capacity Supplemented by Functional Service Provider— Wyeth Business Process Outsourcing Model

In this model the sponsor still retains operational capabilities and the associated maintenance costs in addition to the management of an outsourcing overhead.

Wyeth was challenged to establish a scalable solution to manage a rapidly increasing workload (50% growth in hard copy case record form (CRF) pages in 2004 plus ramp up for electronic data capture (EDC)) for data management workload within the constraints of a fixed staffing headcount. In addition, the driver existed to control or reduce fully loaded processing costs per CRF page and to achieve improvements in performance metrics (e.g., last patient last visit— database lock).

To achieve this, Wyeth implemented an FSP model with Accenture for data management services, a 10-year strategic alliance agreement. Together they reengineered their data management processes and established scalable structures and models using Accenture's global network of delivery centers, leveraging Accenture's 15,000 service personnel across 37 locations where they currently perform business process outsourcing.

All arrangements were structured around performance-based scales where Accenture was compensated on achieving aggressive cost-reduction targets and other key business outcomes. The model was introduced in 2004 associated with around 170 staff being transferred from Wyeth to Accenture.

In the model, Accenture is contracted through penalties and bonuses to continuously improve performance. For example, in 2003, the target was to achieve more than 95% of pages completed imaging and entry within 10 days. By 2007, this is targeted to be within seven days.

The potential advantages of this model are price reductions through process alignment, elimination of activities, and volume discounting and the ability to access less-expensive locations and achieve operational efficiencies.

Resourcing framework for outsourcing drug development Example 3.

Example 3: Full Service Outsourcing (Transitioning into a Mixed Model)— Emerging Pharma

Following an initial simple fee for service arrangement, Addex and Fulcrum put in place an agreement in which Fulcrum provided the majority of Addex's drug development needs followed by a planned transition to a mixed model (6).

Fulcrum provided expertise, business processes, and resources to support early-stage discovery programs targeted to treat diseases of the central nervous system. There was an initial focus on the candidate selection process to ensure the best possible molecules were selected for development. These activities took place in a close working relationship to enable complete transfer of knowledge and responsibilities between the two companies rather than having the process completely in the hands of a contract organization.

Initially, Addex needed support in chemistry, manufacturing and controls (CMC), toxicology, regulatory, clinical, and project management and used Fulcrum's team of experts as required. As the relationship progressed there followed a planned transition in which internal development resources were recruited in a cost-effective manner while projects moved forward at pace.

This allowed Addex to efficiently manage acute and chronic challenges on recruitment and management of high-quality professionals in areas vital for the success of its preclinical and clinical candidate development. In addition, Fulcrum provided solid established processes to audit, contract, and control suppliers' performance and a strong network of validated suppliers that has become critical in moving rapidly during significant stages of development for Addex products.

Addex then established an internal preclinical science group to lead and manage the development of its portfolio and also strengthened its clinical operations to support late-stage products. This was followed by Addex directly contracting and managing several CROs for some aspects of its drug development programs while Fulcrum continued to provide specialists thus supporting CMC and toxicology.

This arrangement enabled the sponsor to take products from powder to proof of concept in 2.5 years and institutionalize processes for translating research into late-stage clinical projects. As a result, Addex's management was able to focus on core activities and deal making plus reduce operational costs by 30% during a three-year period of growth, establishing a portfolio of early- and late-stage products and fundraising.

ENABLING INFRASTRUCTURE AND PROCESSES

A functional-enabling infrastructure supported by clear processes is essential for effective project management of outsourced drug development. This needs to be associated with awareness and training across all the functions and projects. For small companies, this means management must be realistic as to how it can outsource efficiently and focus on those elements where it can have the maximum effect.

Interestingly, it is estimated that many large pharma companies incur significant overhead costs when outsourcing. For example, it is not uncommon for up to 5 sponsor staff to be utilized for every 10 staff from a CRO for the contract duration. This is clearly inefficient and reduces the significant cost and time benefits that should be achievable through outsourcing. It is the experience of the authors that with the right skill sets and processes it is possible to reduce the management or overhead resource to around 10%. This requires "fit–for-purpose" infrastructure, processes, and systems, tailored to the size of the sponsor company and the functions or project work being outsourced. Table 1 summarizes the key elements.

Table 1   Infrastructure, Processes, and Systems for Managing Outsourced Work

Infrastructure, processes, and system	Purpose
Supplier selection process	To ensure suppliers have the desired attributes for the work being contracted out. These attributes will include having the required skill-sets, resources, fiscal stability, track record, and culture. This is a critical step in effective risk management of outsourced drug development.
e-sourcing	To provide a technique for speeding and optimising price negotiations. Can be used as a 'reverse' auction where suppliers are prequalified and then bid down from a preselected price, i.e., e bay in reverse. This works well for commodity services but is an additional step in the sourcing process.
Contract management system employing MSAs plus work order or addendum structures	MSA—To define the common contractual umbrella architecture to ensure consistency, quality, and transactional efficiency. Usually, MSAs cover the following: Definitions, objectives of the relationship, term and duration, service conduct, staff and resources, payment, termination, record keeping and access, confidentiality, intellectual property, indemnification, insurance, limitation of liability, and severance.
	Addendum—To describe the scope of work, customer and supplier responsibilities, deliverables plus cost and time for a given project or process to be performed under the terms of the MSA. It is can also be used as a mechanism to capture and be transparent about deviations from the MSA.
Governance structures	To provide oversight for monitoring and managing performance within projects and across projects. The seniority of staff managing oversight of the "customer–supplier relationship" needs to be fit for purpose according to the complexity of each deal structure. (Fig.1)
	For deals that go beyond tactical outsourcing, the governance structure will often consist of a steering committee of senior individuals from both the customer and the supplier. Under these circumstances the purpose of the governance structure will also be

Table 1 (Continued)

Infrastructure, processes, and system	Purpose
	• to define issue escalation mechanisms.
	• to proactively define measures for relationship success (metrics/KPI, balanced scorecard) and provide a robust and consistent decision-making mechanism where resource decisions can be taken.
	• to take a long-term view of resourcing across projects to align a resource framework and outsourcing strategy with future capability/capacity demands.
Resource planning	To forecast demand and predict cross-project peaks/troughs in resource utilization and enable planning for internal and external resources over time.
Project and financial tracking tools	To manage budgets and track data on actual expenditure, commitments, and any validated negotiated savings. To monitor project progress and provide management with the information required to adjust to any significant changes.
Process for measurement of outcomes, expectations, and deliverables	To drive performance by defining expectations and outcomes at the outset of a project and to describe how these will be measured (metrics).
Quality system and tools	To discharge the responsibilities of the sponsor and ensure outsourced work is compliant with GCP, GLP, GMP, and all relevant external and internal regulations/processes.

Abbreviations: MSA, master service agreement; GCP, Good Clinical Practice; GLP, Good Laboratory Practice; GMP, Good Manufacturing Practice.

SUPPLIER SELECTION

As stated in the table above, effective and efficient supplier selection is important for risk management of outsourcing and therefore warrants a separate section in this chapter. There are a plethora of individual specialist suppliers, niche and "full service" providers, who can enable sponsor companies to outsource the entire drug development process or parts of it. This supplier market is complex and factors in managing this market include services and expertise, costs, quality, contractual and fiscal management, fiscal stability, culture, technology, geographic variability, and future developments, for example, merger and acquisitions.

Supplier selection is therefore a critical process in the project management of outsourcing and effective risk management within a business. If a company gets this wrong then however good its subsequent systems are, the results can range from uncontrolled costs through to product development failure. None of these outcomes are acceptable. However, if the company gets it right then the chances of achieving the benefits of outsourcing increase significantly.

The critical nature of this process should be reflected in a defined and documented supplier selection policy or standard operating procedure (SOP). This process needs to be rigorous and linked to the sponsor company's quality system. Further the policy or SOP should be reviewed and updated regularly on the basis of the experiences and knowledge gained during interactions before, during, and after the management of the supplier selection. This enables continuous improvement in supplier selection and generates intellectual capital.

A supplier selection policy should outline the procedures for the qualification of suppliers and subsequent processes for selection. Expectations need to be applied to all drug development activities on behalf of the sponsor company regarding the applicable good quality practices (GCP, GLP, and Good Manufacturing Practice (GMP)), regulations, and guidelines. Local laws and regulations such as Sarbanes-Oxley should also be applied.

The overall aim of a supplier selection process should be to gather information about the circumstances, competencies, and the relative costs of why a supplier or group of suppliers have been selected to fit a particular project needs. The process consists of several stages. The following list gives examples of a logical and stepwise approach to outsourcing work:

(i)   Define the type of relationship that is required with the supplier, for example, tactical or strategic (Fig. 1) and the scope of work to be outsourced.

(ii)   Select a pool of potential and eligible suppliers either from an in-house or a commercially available database.

(iii)   For new suppliers provide "requests for information" to complete and return with the intention of learning about their business, scope of services, and particular expertise.

(iv)   Based on a positive assessment of the requests for information arrange face to face meetings to confirm cultural and strategic fit, overall expertise, and the services provided.

(v)   At this stage, new suppliers can be audited, a master services agreement (MSA) put in place and they can be added to the database of approved suppliers.

(vi)   Provide a "request for proposal" to a number of selected suppliers (best practice normally is to select three suppliers for cost and capability or capacity choice) and based on the responses, qualification information, and interrogation of bids face-to-face (bid defense) select one provider, agree the deliverables, cost and time for the work being outsourced, and consolidate this information into an addendum to the MSA.

As a variation to the above sequence, value can be added to the process by auditing suppliers specifically against the scope of work to be delivered rather than a general audit looking for GXP (GCP, GLP, GMP) compliance, etc. This is a good example of project managing the risk and maximizing the chances of successful delivery through the selection process.

Good management of outsourcing also demands that if needed, suppliers on a company's database are also deselected according to specific criteria, for example, breach of MSA "for cause," major variances of project-specific milestones and costs, and persistent issues relating to quality.

GOVERNANCE STRUCTURES FOR EFFECTIVE PROJECT MANAGEMENT OF VENDOR/SUPPLIER RELATIONSHIP

Governance structures should have the specific remit and focus to support project delivery and key business goals as opposed to falling into the trap of becoming unstructured and unproductive talking shops. This is best achieved by specifically structuring governance around your sourcing strategy and supply chain framework.

Operational and Executive Governance

Relationship management is an essential part of good governance. Relationships may need to be established to different levels especially where complexity is involved. For example, there is operational governance that can facilitate supplier and sponsor interactions to form single efficient teams and executive governance of the business relationship between sponsor and supplier to try to create and monitor value creation for both parties.

Between the various governance structures, we suggest that specific governance activities, responsibilities, and functions are clearly assigned for the three components discussed in Table 2. This "3P" model will help assist in focusing and prioritizing the actionable areas that can lead to improvement.

Together the operational and executive governance mechanisms should provide an effective support structure by which the pharmaceutical project manager can maintain visibility of the key parameters crucial to the success of their project while not becoming bogged down in non-project-related business issues.

The governance structures become increasingly important when a supplier supports multiple projects across a diverse number of projects or indeed when a project is reliant on a number of suppliers across a complex supply chain, such as described earlier. Over the past few years, focused governance is being formally recognized as a key to improving efficiency and productivity in organizations. Gradually, organizations are moving away from managing each individual project with replicated, inefficient governance and high accompanying overhead to a model of operational responsibilities governed by the project teams. An executive governance mechanism may be a valuable supplement to take on specific cross-project or cross-functional responsibilities and manage the supplier rather than manage everything at the granular project level. Accompanying this change in the industry is a move to the creation of new specific roles to provide focused support to the design, implementation, and management of effective operational and

Table 2 3P Model

Past/retrospective	Present	Prospective
Retrospective analysis and sharing of best practice	Issue escalation forum plus review forum to ensure effective operational issue management	Potential future commitments and opportunity analysis
Learning from past mistakes and successes	Defined measures for success and failure and management against measures	Future success measures for both parties to optimize value for both parties
	Metrics and KPIs: relationship, quality, cost, risk, time, efficiency, and productivity	
	Financial oversight (overall commitments and actual expenditures)	Open view of any future impacts on business model either party if likely to effect relationship (change in strategic direction, merger/acquisition)
	Project management oversight	
	Risk management	Risk management

Abbreviation: KPI, key performance indicators.

executive governance such as supply chain managers, vendor relations managers, supplier governance leads, and business development executives.

A good governance model should add quantifiable value to both parties and serve to support and strengthen the overall relationship desired by both parties aiding transparency and maximizing productivity. Like many things, there will be a range of governance mechanisms available and one should select the most appropriate for the individual circumstances.

In case of ad hoc relationships with low-expenditure and noncritical work, it should be recognized that governance may be relatively informal. In these circumstances, it may occur almost entirely at operational levels through operational management teams or joint project teams with issue escalation through line management routes, with suppliers working internationally and across supply chains and/or projects with sponsors, though this will be inefficient unless supported by an overarching executive governance umbrella. Such an executive team must be empowered and senior enough to be able to take the tough decisions and provide leadership within both organizations. The threshold at which it becomes efficient to affect a strategic governance framework and make these investments is a management decision that ultimately should be driven by productivity and efficiency metric data such as the number and types of issues detected, time lines, cost, and resource overhead.

Metrics, Performance, and Balanced Scorecards

Together metrics and key performance indicators (KPIs) can aid organizations to manage project delivery and anticipate and manage risk. The two are often confused but should be differentiated as they serve separate purposes.

KPIs are those performance indicators that are directly linked to the strategic outsourcing objectives. KPIs are often confused with "metrics"; the main distinction is that KPIs can be considered as either a key indicator of success or the "sum" of a number of metrics. Examples of KPIs could be achievement of project targets, efficiency, or productivity.

Metrics are detailed measures of various aspects of performance. Usually, metrics measure individual process steps that are done repeatedly or intermediate outcomes of a process. Examples of clinical metrics could be time from first patient enrolled to last patient enrolled, number audit findings, and cost per patient.

It is recommended also that with any relationship both parties define some key metrics to measure the success or failure of a relationship. These may be project related but could also take into account other areas. Relationship metrics are of particular value and increased relevance with the more strategic partnership relationships such as copromotion, codevelopment, or licensing-type arrangements. Good metrics and KPIs along with effective governance structured around a clear sourcing and supply chain strategy provide strong support for organizational change from tactical risk-management practices to more strategic management structures, which will bring accompanying efficiencies and productivity gains. Implementing a directional change in sourcing strategy without the means to measure success or failure is unlikely to achieve your desired outcome. Often it takes two to three years to refine and align strategy and for the operational components to achieve the desired outcomes. Without a good toolkit to measure the cause and effect, refinement and fine-tuning will be frustrating and difficult. Strategic risk management combined with effective governance is a powerful combination to achieve process optimization and supply chain efficiency and productivity and value creation. A simple progressive model used to manage risk is shown in Table 3.

The starting point for building any metrics is to consider the risk-management model being employed to support your sourcing strategy. With a complex supply chain the likelihood is that governance will be focused on process and multiple functions and projects with individual suppliers.

Key metrics (Fig. 4) can be designed as indicators of efficiency and productivity and generally aid operational governance structures to monitor delivery and utilization of resources.

Table 3 Risk Management—Five Progressive Models to Manage Risk

Crisis management	Risks are not addressed until they create problems either because management is not aware of the risks or has inaccurately estimated their probability of occurring. Addresses existing problems, can be exciting but causes burnout. It is a fix on failure approach.	Tactical
Risk management	Introduction of risk concepts to reduce probability and consequences, e.g., contingency planning, consequences, and what if scenarios.	
Prevention	Shift of risk management from individual manager to team activity. Rather than avoidance of risk move to eliminate and avoid root causes. It is a move from reactive to proactive risk management.	
Anticipate	Move from subjective to quantitative risk management using metrics to anticipate failures and predict future events. Anticipated problems are avoided through early prioritized corrective actions.	
Opportunity	Positive version of risk management used to innovate and shape future states. Uses perception of risk as chances to save money or do better than planned.	Strategic

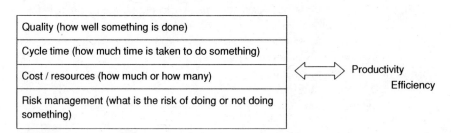

Quality (how well something is done)

Cycle time (how much time is taken to do something)

Cost / resources (how much or how many)   Productivity
                                                  Efficiency
Risk management (what is the risk of doing or not doing something)

Figure 4 Key metrics.

KPIs by contracts are measures that enable senior management to maintain a comprehensive overview of the business and effectiveness of the overall sourcing strategy and supply chain in question. They may include financial and nonfinancial data possibly generated from internal and externals metric data. One way of presenting and reviewing such data is through the use of balanced scorecards.

Balanced Scorecards

Metrics can be rolled up into KPIs. KPIs can then be consolidated within a balanced scorecard to achieve a visual indication of key performance. Dependant upon the outcome desired, individual parameters could be weighted to reflect priority and desired behaviors.

(i) Traffic Light Systems

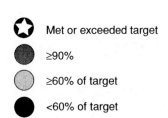

⭐	Met or exceeded target
⬤	≥90%
◯	≥60% of target
⬤	<60% of target

(ii) Trend Indicators

+-	Result increasing, Performance deteriorating
--	Result decreasing, Performance deteriorating
++	Result increasing, Performance improving
-+	Result increasing, Performance improving
0	No change since last result or no data available to calculate trend

Figure 5 Ways to report metrics.

To illustrate this for a sourcing strategy, the suggested KPIs could be

- service, delivery, and quality,
- customer and supplier relationships,
- contract and cost management, and
- innovation and learning.

Within each area, the KPI would be a set of metrics that are regularly scored. As far as possible, these metrics should be objective and realistic, i.e., capable of being measured. These scorecards, with their underlying metric data and interpretation, can then be used to provide actionable results for project managers and senior management. They are the instrument panel to oversee overall performance but capable of interrogation to identify the causation of failure or quantify and trend success. Typical mechanisms used to report status of metric information on scorecards are shown in Figure 5.

The main benefits of using a balanced scorecard are that it

- allows performance measurement from a number of different aspects, all of which contribute to overall performance.
- illustrates target results and trends against strategic business goals.
- avoids the risk of "management by anecdote"—performance assessment is based on concrete data and the contribution of all parties to that performance can be evaluated.

Table 4   Recommendations When Using Balanced Scorecards

Dos	Don'ts
• Use the KPI report on a regular basis within a management team forum to ○ understand variations to expected performance and what is driving them, ○ resolve any issues to alleviate future risks and improve performance and capabilities, and ○ learn from past performances and celebrate success.	• Do not look for whom to blame when there is a "red light" as this serves as an early warning indicator. Instead, leverage the team to find creative ways of resolving issues before they have an impact on performance.
• Review your KPIs over time to ensure that they drive the appropriate behaviors in line with your strategic goals.	• Do not relate "red light" with punishment. If people associate "red light" with punishment, in time, no red lights will be reported and the scorecard will not act as an early warning system.
• Ensure that the scorecard drives an *action* orientation at all times.	• Do not hold people accountable for targets that they cannot influence.
	• Do not focus solely on past performance—pay at least as much attention to indicators that reflect future performance.

Abbreviations: KPI, key performance indicators.

- provides a consistent framework for assessing performance—a "level playing field"—wherever multiple suppliers are used.
- provides a forum for constructive, objective feedback and facilitates goal setting for future performance.

The recommendations to be considered when using balanced scorecards are discussed in Table 4.

CONCLUSION

A variety of business models, processes, and tools for operating and managing outsourced drug development have been described in this chapter. These can provide the necessary framework and rigor for the effective project management of outsourced drug development. However, managers, tools, and processes will need to be increasingly sophisticated as the management of drug development programs is set to become even more complex due to increasing competition and regulation. Future challenges include the following:

1. *Investor expectations of improved capital efficiency in product development*
   - Emerging pharma and biotech companies can no longer build expensive infrastructure during early finance rounds and must contract out extensively. Indeed, all companies need to look for competitive advantage beyond their core competencies increasing the need for effective project management of complex, outsourced, multidisciplinary projects. Such programs go way beyond the outsourcing of clinical or preclinical studies and can encompass all the disciplines of drug development.
2. *Changing and ever more stringent regulation*
   - The introduction of ICH-GCP within the United States, Japan, and Europe, via the Clinical Trials Directive 2001/2002 in Europe, has led to an increasingly regulated environment. Recently, the recommendations resulting from the disastrous phase 1 clinical study on Tegenero's monoclonal antibody, TGN 1412 will only add to this for innovative, new medicines. Further, this clinical study highlights the challenges of managing outsourced development plus the need for rigor to ensure patient safety and compliance.
3. *The emergence of the "mega trial" phenomenon*
   - Sponsor companies continue to look for ways to reduce the cost of developing new medicines through efficiency and productivity gains. As a result, late-stage development programs tend to focus on fewer clinical trials per submission with more patients per trial resulting in the so-called global registration mega trial. Such programs are usually designed with multiple end points and sufficient statistical power to demonstrate phase 3 safety within a minimal number of trials. This is time and cost efficient since a small number of mega trails can be completed more quickly than having to conduct a larger number of single end point trials yet still generate sufficient regulatory data for submission. Clearly, the scale of this approach again increases the complexity and scope of project management and the need for effective management of risk to ensure delivery.

These examples show that the role of project management and project managers is being redefined from conducting simple "in-house" projects to now include management of complex projects, which contain multiple disciplines and use both internal and external resources (7). Looking forward, the role of the pharmaceutical project manager will continue to grow and the skills—tools plus processes—that they employ will be pivotal to the future success of pharmaceutical biotech companies and suppliers alike.

REFERENCES

1. Chaturvedi S. Outsourcing in the Pharmaceutical Industry. Available at www.bionity.com/articles/e/49803; 2007.
2. Martorelli, MA. Growth in the outsourcing sector set to continue. Scrip 100 2006:36.

3. Tufts Center for the Study of Drug Development News and Events. CROs usage associated with faster drug development speed at comparable quality. Available at http://csdd.tufts.edu/Newsevents/News Article. Accessed on January 23, 2006.
4. Tufts Center for the Study of Drug Development. CRO contribution to drug development is substantial and growing globally. Tufts CSDD Impact Report, 2006; Volume 8, No. 1.
5. Morgan R, Bravard JL. Smarter Outsourcing: An Executive Guide to Managing Successful Relationships, FT Prentice Hall, Great Britain, 2006.
6. Mutel V, Court JP. Collaborations from candidate to proof of concept. Abstract from SciPharm Conference, Edinburgh, 2006.
7. Vogel JR, Getz KA. Successful Outsourcing of Clinical Drug Developments. BioExecutive International June 2006 Supplement Series, pp. 30–38.

10

The Project Management Function

Tony Kennedy
Trigen Ltd., London, U.K.

INTRODUCTION

This chapter is about "pharmaceutical project management" as a function. It discusses the roles and responsibilities of the function and how it can be organized. The main types of jobs within the function are described and the skills and competencies needed reviewed. In many companies, the project management group plays a role in supporting the pharma organization and particularly the development organization. This may include the organization of portfolio review meetings and performance setting and appraisal for project teams and providing support for key management oversight committees. In addition, the function is often charged with the leadership of initiatives to improve the drug development processes. The precise structure of a project management group varies considerably between companies both in remit, reporting line and the scope of responsibilities given to staff. Job titles vary a lot. The size of a company also is an important factor in determining the needs. Big pharma companies not only need project management at the individual project level but also need to have functional project management capabilities to effectively manage large portfolios. This chapter will describe the evolution of project management in the pharmaceutical industry over the past 25 years. It will highlight the potential contributions that project management can make to manage effectively what will always be an immensely challenging enterprise—making medicines from molecules.

EVOLUTION OF THE PHARMACEUTICAL PROJECT
MANAGEMENT FUNCTION

Taking drugs from their discovery through development to registration and launch is a complex, lengthy, multidisciplinary endeavour. The enterprise is highly risky and consumes substantial resources. Companies large and small have recognized the need to establish effective management processes to progress projects to agreed development plans and to budget. Organization structure and organizational process clearly differ significantly between companies. Larger pharma companies from the 1970/80s progressively established central project management groups and some, though not all, decided to place responsibility for the leadership and management of the international projects within such groups. This represented a departure from earlier management approaches that had either had a development committee attempting to manage projects directly or charged disciplinary experts with a leadership responsibility. Often a discovery senior scientist would lead an early phase project and a senior clinician take on leadership for the project when it entered patient trials.

In the larger pharma companies, the very size of the development portfolio meant that development committees could not realistically manage projects directly. Moreover, it was recognized that there was a need for greater consistency in approach to managing projects and in gathering project-related data to make sense of a portfolio view. In addition, senior management was under increasing pressure to accelerate the pace of drug development, which was often very protracted. In part, this was because of the inefficiencies within the pharma industry itself. However, it was also compounded by the lengthy regulatory approval times. The industry response was in most cases to introduce some form of project management within development. Over the period of the 1980s and 1990s, an increasing number of people took up full time positions in project management. In addition, companies were increasingly concerned to benchmark their performances against rival companies. Some companies turned to the big management consultancy firms to help them improve development processes. Invariably, the internal project management groups because of their acquired "big picture" view of development became central players in process improvement projects. Management also was keen to explore outsourcing initiatives to test whether internal functions were as efficient, cost effective, and quick as outside best practice. Some innovative experiments were run. As one example, Roche spanned out a virtual development company Protodigm to test the virtual development model. As another example, Abbott threw the ball to their project management giving them budget responsibility and freedom to allocate work contracts.

So, the industry project management roles and responsibilities differed substantially between true "business within a business" groups charged with successful delivery of projects and given considerable freedom of action and, at the other extreme, decorative "project management" nameplates on doors but no real change in drug development management practice.

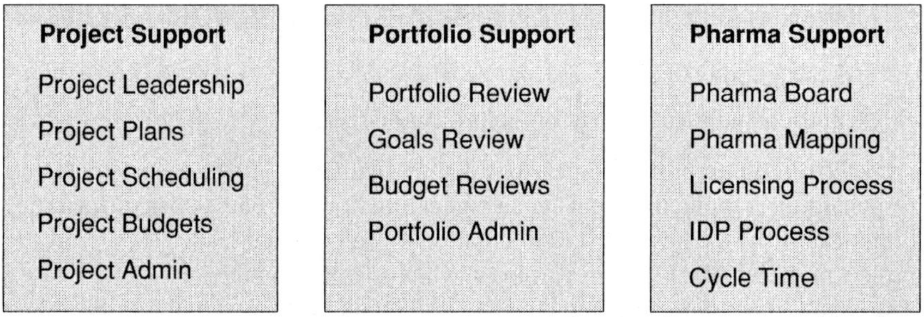

Project Support	Portfolio Support	Pharma Support
Project Leadership	Portfolio Review	Pharma Board
Project Plans	Goals Review	Pharma Mapping
Project Scheduling	Budget Reviews	Licensing Process
Project Budgets	Portfolio Admin	IDP Process
Project Admin		Cycle Time

Figure 1 The project management function. *Abbreviation*: IDP, integrated development plan.

Over this period, big changes were occurring outside the pharma companies. The wealth of the big companies with blockbuster products meant that huge sums of money were pumped into drug development and the market responded. Contract research came of age and with it came both a sharpening of practice and an operational flexibility that suited a mixed sourcing solution for pharma companies. Effective Contract Research Organization (CRO) project management played a key role in achieving this.

Within pharma companies, another challenge was where to place a project management function within the organizational reporting lines. Some people were adamant that it had to report directly to the CEO or it would be "toothless." Others were equally persuaded that it must report to the head of development. Another view was that it should report to the head of central marketing so that it would operate with a business ethos rather than a technical ethos. Discovery was also very keen to implement project management capability. In practice, all these options were implemented in different companies and, over the years, "migrations" in line reporting occurred. From a company perspective, the most important point was that smart people were devoting their working lives to the task of project management.

In summary, during the past 25 years the role of project management has evolved within the Industry. In the bigger companies, the project management function has contributed in three areas—providing support for individual projects, supporting portfolio management, and playing an important role in improving the way pharma brings medicines to market. Figure 1 illustrates these roles. In the text that follows, the roles themselves will be further described. The skills and competencies needed to perform theses roles will be considered. In addition, attention will be given to how these skills can be acquired.

PROJECT SUPPORT

The following activities need to be competently performed to manage projects:

• Leadership of projects

- Management of projects
- Creation of the development plans
- Scheduling of the project
- Definition and management of the project budget

While different companies will define distinctive job titles and roles and responsibilities for their project management function, there are two main job types often established. These are the international project team leader (IPL) and the project manager (PM). "Hybrid" roles in which elements of the job types are fused also exist. Sometimes, the job incumbent still retains some residual line discipline responsibility. Because of this variety in job titles, it is important to look beyond the title in any organization and get the sense of what actually has to be done.

International Project Leader

The IPL's role is to provide leadership to the international project team (IPT) and to report to the committee that manages the development portfolio, for example, the product development committee (PDC). The position is a senior one reflecting the broad responsibility and the knowledge and experience required to do the job. It is worth noting that the IPL may be managing a project over potentially a three to four years' duration during which perhaps £100 million to £200 million or more will be spent deploying the resources of hundreds of internal and external staff.

To fulfill the role, the job holder needs the following qualities:

- excellent general management competency,
- strong drug development knowledge, and
- a broad familiarity with project management skills.

The job is a demanding one requiring the incumbent to have the intellectual ability to deal with complexity and to work with the team specialists to create a far-sighted strategy and plan for the project. It is important to have the vision to rise above the technical elements to recognize the essential value proposition of the project and how that needs to be shaped into a clear product definition. IPT core team members will be from discovery, preclinical development, clinical development, manufacturing, regulatory, and marketing teams. The core team is supported by subteams (see chap. 1). A key contribution of an effective IPL is to harness the expertise within and beyond the team to select the right development strategy for the project. Operationally, the IPT typically meets monthly to review the results from completed studies and to agree forward plans. The IPL plays a key role in ensuring that new issues arising are put into an appropriate perspective and that actions to resolve the issues are promptly defined. The IPL plays the principal role in communicating from the IPT to the PDC and vice versa. The IPL working with the core IPT will define the annual goals for the IPT that will be set into the project plan and budget. The IPL will be charged with delivery of the

PDC-sanctioned project plan to time, cost, and quality. Because projects rarely go according to plan, the IPL generally will need to revert to the PDC to gain sanction for contingency actions and associated deviation approvals for budgets and schedule. The people management aspects of the job are very important. The IPT and the PDC look to the IPL to make good judgment. Examples include recognizing that an IPT member is unable to provide the needed expertise to the team (for a variety of possible reasons) and taking action to resolve the problem and also showing maturity and clear thinking at PDC when recommending actions to resolve project issues. For high-priority projects, the IPL role invariably is stressful. Some very capable people realize pretty soon that it is not meant for them.

What management attributes should an IPL have? Integrative analytical skills are important because many project issues are cross-disciplinary. Interpersonal skills are critical to the role. Typically, the phrases that are cited in job specifications include "independent minded, courageous, energetic, tenacious, motivating, practical, entrepreneurial, good judgment, communicator, personable, direct, and honest." Most of us recognize the sort of people these words attempt to describe.

Drug development skills are also highly important to the IPL. An understanding of the strategic aspects of drug development is essential. Thus, product-profile setting to ensure that market intent is matched in the label intent and that the development plan provides the data to achieve both. It is important that clear decision points are established to ensure that further investment in the project can be justified or that an early termination decision is made. A broad understanding of the scope of the development activities and how they fit together is also important. Development "functions" try to support the project team by sending experienced representatives to the IPT. As issues arise, informal discussion between function head and the IPL may be needed from time to time to "clear the air" with the team representative from the function participating. The IPL should have a good understanding of pharmaceutical project management skills including project planning and budgeting techniques to have the confidence to challenge assumptions on the project schedule and variations in the project expenditure. The IPL for major projects generally will have the support of one or more PMs depending on the scale of the project workload. The IPL will not have the detailed knowledge and expertise that the PM brings to their work. The IPL needs to focus on project strategy while the day-to-day project management is driven by able PMs; it is truly a project management "team" effort that powers good drug development.

It is perhaps not surprising that because the scope of the IPL job is broad and demanding it is seen as a "test bed" job for senior managers destined to move on to leadership roles within pharma functions or as country managers. After three to four years as an IPL, the incumbent will certainly understand a great deal more about the nature of the business of new drug development and their own company's way of doing things.

Project Manager

The PM plays a key operational role in driving the project forward. Big projects in late development phase are extremely busy enterprises. The IPT must focus on the top-level plan while it is in the subteams that the operational project management occurs. Thus, there will be very active preclinical, clinical, Chemistry, Manufacturing Controls (CMC), regulatory, and marketing subteams. Many functions themselves have dedicated PMs to manage and coordinate the work. The central project management group PMs play a key interface role between the IPT and subteams working with both the function IPT lead (e.g., clinical team leader) and PMs from the function. In this way, the IPT strategy and plan is "joined up" with functional plans and potential mismatch between the two recognized quickly and resolved. For some scientists moving from functional management positions, the PM position is the point of entry into project management. The chance to work as a PM on a busy project provides a great opportunity to learn on the job. Thereafter, there is the chance to lead and manage one of the many smaller projects, which might be an early phase project or perhaps a discrete life cycle project such as new formulation development. Such assignments give the incumbent and the company an opportunity to assess the caliber and potential of the PM to progress to an IPL position.

The PM plays a key role within the project management function and within the IPT by establishing and maintaining the project schedule and budget. The PM works closely with other project management staff including other PMs and the IPL and also with the functional PMs, the finance group, and periodically the portfolio management group. The PM needs to be "in the loop" so that any changes in the project strategy and plan are rapidly reflected in the project schedule and budget. The planning interface between project teams and functions is particularly critical. Central project plans often "wrap up" detailed activities and costs. Synchrony in changes to functional and central plans is important to avoid disparity when budgets are viewed from line and project portfolio perspectives.

PMs may be recruited from company staff working in scientific functional departments or from other groups such as finance and accounting. There is a case to be made for having a mix of staff from scientific and finance backgrounds because of the interfaces with both the areas.

An able PM makes a real contribution to IPT and to the company. The annual budget-setting process is invariably followed by significant changes within a project. As a result, some activities are stopped and others expanded. Fleet footwork is needed to maintain an accurate and up-to-date picture for time and budget. Despite the best of "process optimization," it is often the good working relationships and initiative of the PM that allows a clear current picture to be shown.

To fulfill the role, the PM needs the following qualities:

- good people skills,
- good general management skills,

- strong drug development competency, and
- strong project management competency.

Evidence for good general management skills should be sought during the recruitment of the PM. It is one reason why many PM positions are filled internally on "the devil you know" principle. Additionally, companies are keen to retain talent and realize that some able functional scientific managers want to advance their career ambitions beyond the function and may have potential to be good general managers. While on-the-job skills acquisition is important, good training in drug development and project management is critical to get the best performance from the PM. Therefore, companies need to invest in training to bring talented scientific managers to a high level in drug development competency. Good interpersonal skills are essential to engender cooperation and flow of information between disciplines.

Activities to Support the Project

Project Team Management

There are a number of simple practices that can be followed to ensure that project teams run effectively. The work of the project team is essentially in three phases: set up, implementation, and review or more concisely "plan, do, check." The development of a drug from discovery through development to the market and during life cycle management is really a series of projects that sit beneath an overall strategic plan, which charts the strategic intent and the path to market (Fig. 2). The nearer term plan is specified at a detail level to allow activities to be planned and scheduled and an integrated development plan (IDP) is created to frame an investment proposal for management sanction.

The planning phase includes the selection of the target indication, the development strategy, and the operational plan for the investment phase ahead. This is an intensive phase of work for the project team. They will use the tools described in chapter 1 such as the target product profile (TPP) and IDP template to analyze and integrate the information on the project. The core team meets regularly to review the draft IDP. The project team leader (PTL) and PM play a driving role to ensure that the IDP comes together as a coherent and concise document. Risk assessment and contingency plans should be included. As appropriate, an alternative scenario can be offered if in the planning stage some potential advantages to "plan B" were recognized. With the approval of the IDP the team moves into the "do" phase. Project team meetings are held periodically to review the progress of the project against the plan and address issues that inevitably will arise seeking a resolution that keeps the project as closely to plan as is possible. Deviations from the approved plan need to be promptly notified to the oversight PDC committee to ensure that an investment mandate remains in place.

Project team meetings can usually be sensibly scheduled on a monthly basis for a rolling six-month calendar. There is real benefit in getting into a disciplined

The strategic plan: Tracing the path to market

Investment cycles and project plans

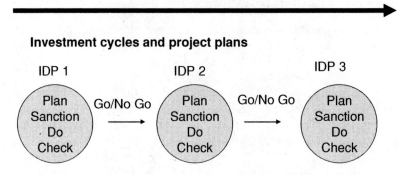

Development of a drug from discovery to market and through life cycle management is a series of projects for which investment must be justified.

Figure 2 Strategic plans and project plans.

rhythm with good agenda setting and its precirculation before the meeting to allow team members to prepare properly. This preparation should ensure that the line function has discussed team issues thoroughly from a line perspective so that the team representative comes to the project team meeting with a mature position. The agenda itself will often be put together by the PM having talked to the project team members to highlight issues that need to be discussed. Usually, the agenda has three components. Firstly, the status updates by the line functions describing the work they have conducted. This is most efficiently handled by the line functions sending in a concise summary to the PM who collates the material and circulates it to the team prior to the meeting. Specific items from this "work progress report" can then be discussed on an exception basis. Secondly, issues that have arisen need to be reviewed by the team and proposed resolution actions approved. The third element is for the team to check whether there have been any significant deviations from plan over the past month and whether there is anything that jeopardizes the planned and scheduled activities looking forward.

The IPL and the PM will refine the agenda to assign priority, allocate appropriate time for items, and agree upon the team members who would be given the responsibilities. It is important that "issues" come to the project team having been discussed by a relevant team subgroup with a recommendation for resolution. Individual companies often have their preferred systems for issue analysis and decision making. The "STP" (situation, target, proposal) works well. For more complex challenges the full Kepner-Tregoe process is valuable.

The IPL needs to actively steer the agenda and the discussion. It is valuable to have open team discussion of STPs to make sure that the case for the proposed action is robust and that alternative solutions have been carefully considered. On some occasions, the IPL will recognize that the discussion needs to be closed down because it has become apparent that critical information has not been factored into an STP or perhaps the team does not have the needed specific expertise. In these circumstances, a follow up subgroup meeting needs to be actioned, perhaps bringing in additional expertise.

Project team meeting (PTM) documentation needs to be concise. The minutes need to be focused on the issues and the actions (what, who, when). It is good practice to get out an "actions summary" list within a day of the meeting. STPs and work progress summary reports can efficiently be attached as appendices to minutes and can serve to reduce the text in the minutes. There are different schools of thought on minutes. The "transcript" minutes style "Fred said . . . then Dick said . . ." has few advocates. The "skeleton" style "action1, action2, action3" has popular following. The author favors minutes in which a reader can readily find an adequate definition of the issue, the resolution action itself, and the team endorsed rationale for the action. The sometimes convoluted track that took the team to its conclusion can usefully be omitted. The purpose of recording minutes is to provide the team and the broader organization with an adequate record of the progression of the project and the changes to the original plan and why they were made. The work of the team must be effectively communicated. The circulation of minutes to senior management and line functions is one vehicle. In addition, team representatives need to brief their line managers and the proactive IPL will discuss issues with relevant senior managers. Figure 3 summarizes project team meeting management.

The third phase of the project team work is the "check" phase in which the team reviews whether the plan was successfully delivered or not and whether there is a basis for recommending the further progression of the project. Chapter 1 discussed the importance of the careful review of project data at phase-transition points. The team needs to review the data now available at the end of this phase of development and decide whether to recommend progression of the project. The tools highlighted in chapter 1 (big 5 questions and the TPP) help the team in this deliberation. The team will present a recommendation to the PDC and gain sanction to create the next phase IDP.

Computerized Project Planning

Chapter 3 describes how project plans are established and how they relate to other types of project information. External training programs are offered by a number of companies in project planning with different planning software. Within the larger pharma companies, different planning systems often coexist with central project management running one type of software and functional groups using different systems. Enterprisewide planning systems are used in some companies. As highlighted by Les Rose in chapter 6, there are multiple levels that project activities can be planned at. The level of detail needs to be relevant to the user group to track and monitor progress and to manage resource allocation.

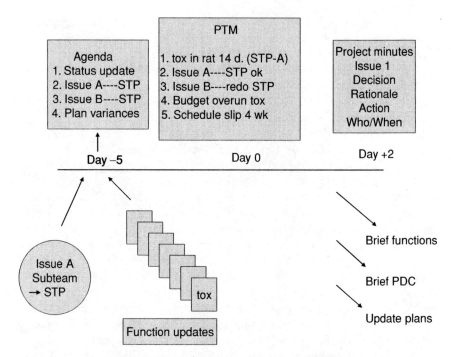

Figure 3 PTM cycle. *Abbreviations*: PTM, project team meeting; STP, situation, target, proposal; PDC, product development committee.

Project Budgeting

Establishing and maintaining project budgets is a challenging task. Project plans frequently change during a year with new activities being undertaken and planned activities not being progressed. Cost estimates for studies, particularly clinical, often have to be revised in light of feasibility studies or to address the need to speed enrollment by increasing resources for the trial. Maintaining a current budget that accurately reflects anticipated costs therefore is a continuous activity. The PM spends a lot of time in contact with colleagues in the major line functions adapting and revising budgets and checking on whether planned expenditure has actually occurred. While there is an annual cycle for budget setting, it is sensible for quarterly budget updates across the portfolio. As might be expected from the dynamics of a steady-state portfolio, while costs of individual projects have a tendency to rise, the high attrition rate means that some projects fail and planned activities do not happen. It is very important to recognize the scale of committed costs on failed projects because it is often mistakenly assumed by management that there is a larger "piggy bank" of money available to switch from failed to new projects than is the case.

PORTFOLIO SUPPORT

The following key activities are needed to effectively manage the portfolio:

- PDC administrative support
- Goal setting and review
- Budget review
- Portfolio administration

Central Project Management Portfolio Group

A central project management portfolio group is given the responsibility to support the portfolio review process, the goal-setting process, and the development planning guidelines. The group will periodically establish cross-functional teams to improve specific project team processes as requested by the management. The group usually is staffed by highly experienced IPL and PM staff and also act as a support group to the global Head of project management. In some big pharma companies, the development portfolio is of such a size that it is broken up in therapeutic areas. The management of the therapeutic area portfolio can then be assigned to a project management cluster reporting to a therapeutic area head.

Product Development Committee Support

The PDC in a large company is extremely busy and needs to work very efficiently to cover its review and decision-making responsibilities. It needs good support to achieve this. Information overload is a real issue. Therefore, the input materials to the committee need to be concise, accurate, and well focused. The administrative support to the PDC is quite demanding. For the purposes of this discussion, the PDC is the committee that is chaired by the head of the pharmaceutical division (which manages the mid- to late-phase development portfolio and products in the market with active central life cycle investments). At the monthly PDC meetings, the bulk of the agenda is generally given over to specific project team presentations requesting approvals for development strategies and plans and the commitment of resources. In addition, cross-portfolio deviations from plan are discussed. These include budgetary deviations, changes in project schedules (usually slippage), and new findings affecting the attainability of the TPP. The agenda preparation and the minuting of the meeting typically will be the responsibility of project management as will be the coordination of the input documentation. The project management portfolio group can usefully help IPLs with presentation preparations. The group may have developed PDC presentation guidelines. Standardization of presentations appreciably helps PDC efficiency.

Portfolio Review and Asset Valuation Process

Chapter 2 described, in some detail, the techniques that can be used in portfolio management. Chapter 1 highlighted the dynamic state of a portfolio because of the high attrition rates for projects and made the point that, typically, the majority of projects will be at an early phase such as preclinical or phase 1. Most companies carry out periodic portfolio reviews and try to standardize the project "input data" for review. The objective of the review should be to confirm that the project assumptions on which specific investments have been made remain valid and that the resources planned to be devoted to the project are appropriate. These meetings are valuable if well planned and run. There are sometimes surprises revealed through the review. These may include the revelation that substantial development resources do not appear to be allocated to defined projects ("What on earth are your people doing?"), that key project assumptions are invalid ("So, in essence, we are two years later with inferior market differentiation, did I get that right?"), or that there is a pharmaceutical "limbo" with parked projects because of an inability to take decisions but a willingness to defer. Companies develop their own specific systems for the review. In one company, an electronic voting system was implemented by project management to try to improve the quality of decision making. In part, the intent was to achieve a more balanced assessment of projects because invariably one or two senior panel members tended to dominate the discussion and a "fall-in-line" voting behavior was consistently observed at decision time. With this voting system in place, nobody knew who was voting for what and the voting "scores" for a variety of project parameters came on screen for the panel to view (e.g., level of development risk, scale of commercial attractiveness). For most projects, the voting outcomes were generally fairly predictable. However, of greater interest were the 10% to 20% of projects for which wild voting swings were evident. These projects then became the focus of discussion to try to understand the variance. In many instances, misunderstandings about the project assumptions were the root cause of the difference. For example, the commercial attractiveness of a project may have been judged low by some panel members because the product profile was not better on efficacy than a well-established marketed product. However, the commercial team had determined through market research that substitution would be readily achieved because of other limitations of the marketed product, which clearly did not satisfy existing customers.

Over a period of years, there is a tendency for portfolio review meetings to become increasingly cumbersome and unwieldy as each year some additional analysis is bolted on. A periodic "spring cleaning" of the process is needed and a back to basics approach makes good sense. In particular, the level of detail and the extent of the data to be reviewed for the "early portfolio" and the "mid–late portfolio" differ and a lighter touch is required for the former.

Goal Setting and Goals Review Process

Goal setting is a fact of life in most companies in one form or another. There are some clear benefits to a project team setting goals. The process does invite team members to identify their most important project objectives and the exercise generally ensures all team members understand their contribution to achieving the objectives. The specific process followed for goal setting differs significantly between companies. In some, it is a dominating process that is strongly linked to financial reward. One example of the process requests teams to identify three to five specific goals for the year ahead. The goals are specifically defined in such a way as to avoid ambiguity and to allow a "clean" assessment of success or failure to achieve the goal. One year on, at the goals review meeting, the team presents their own assessment of goal achievement for the review panel to approve. Team "goal scores" are calculated. The review panel then has the more difficult task of "calibrating" the score, given their knowledge of the environment. Did team B fail to achieve a registration target through incompetent planning and execution or were there organizational or regulatory agency problems that made the task impossible? An undoubted benefit of the review is that it can serve to detect systemic organizational defects. For example, failure to meet registration dossier submission deadlines for several projects may reflect either inadequate resources in specific departments, inept management, and failure to prioritize or failure to deliver by functional departments. Follow-up review is important. Good judgment and common sense need to be applied if the goals system is to provide overall benefit to a company. It is very demotivating for teams who do not achieve their goals to be heavily penalized if the reasons for failure were completely beyond their control. Another thing to be watched is the parity of performance challenge in the goals set by different teams. Some teams "play the system" by advancing very modest goals while others fly too close to the sun. The review meeting that assesses goal achievements can also be used to assess goal setting for the next year. Management needs to weigh the proposed goals to ensure that the level of challenge is appropriate and realistic.

PHARMA SUPPORT

The following key activities are needed to effectively support the broader pharma organization:

- Pharma mapping
- Licensing and due-diligence process improvement
- Integrated development plan process improvement
- Cycle time reduction process improvement

These activities will be described in more detail.

Pharma Mapping

Put simply, "pharma mapping" is providing a description of the pharma organization and how it works to its people. It seems a pretty obvious thing to do but often it does not happen. Project management's helicopter view makes it an ideal group to drive this type of initiative and it can work usefully with a communications group to produce impactful "products" that can be broadly shared. Mapping can

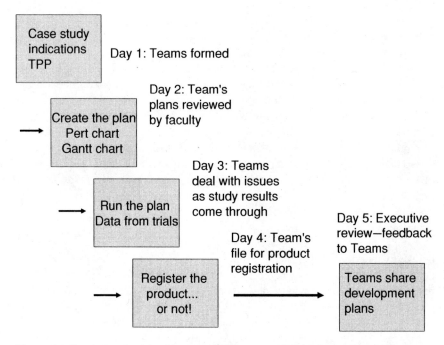

Figure 4   Simulating drug development. *Abbreviation*: TPP, target product profile.

be done at two different levels both of which are valuable. The higher-level "product" can be a brochure that outlines the structure of pharma and its key activities and responsibilities. The role of line functions, project teams, and oversight committees are described. Acronyms and strange function codes are simply explained. The mission and objectives of the company are clearly stated. New starters and those working in the company for many years value this effort to give them a better understanding of their business and their role in it. The mapping can also be taken to a higher granularity that describes the interrelationship of the major functional activities and information flows during the development and market introduction of a product. This can be visually mapped and supported by process description that can be particularly valuable in achieving a greater recognition of the interrelationship between technical, regulatory, and commercial functions and the nature of the information needed at key times in the development cycle. It can bind together functional processes to the broader pharma game plan.

Licensing and Due-Diligence Process

The licensing and due-diligence process is a critical organization competency for pharma companies. There is intense competition between pharma companies to license in promising development projects. The licensing company in such a situation weighs a number of factors in deciding with whom to transact. These factors include the relative attractiveness of deal terms and flexibility to accommodate the licensee strategic objectives (e.g., a wish to codevelop). In addition, the competency and commitment of the in-licensing company will be evident in the way it interacts from initial business group contact through the due-diligence process to deal completion. Speed, efficiency, competency, professionalism, clarity, and integrity are hallmark qualities that will be recognized and can affect partner choice. The licensing process demands that business, technical, and scientific groups work effectively together and know their roles and when to hand them off to others. Project management groups working with business licensing have played a role in defining licensing best practice so that the start to finish process is mapped, products are defined, and performance standards made explicit. These materials are then available for training the many individuals who will be called upon over time to be involved in licensing.

The Integrated Project Plan Process

In chapter 1, the objective and contents of the IDP was described. Project management generally takes a lead in building template plans working with the key functional groups to ensure that the right information is captured at an appropriate level and that the separate, more detailed functional plans (e.g., market launch plans) "mesh" with the IDP. The IDP content may usefully be adjusted to be fit for purpose for the stage of development. The pharma mapping initiative will provide specific examples of information needed for IDP approval at later phase-transition points.

Cycle Time Reduction—Generic Plans

Many medium- and large-sized pharma companies have invested in process improvement projects focused upon reducing development time and increasing the efficiency of development processes. In some cases, these projects have been run in conjunction with consultancy groups. Project management is well positioned to drive this initiative. This can readily be achieved with the establishment of a cross-functional team bringing together the most experienced functional managers with the best project management staff. By bringing together the expertise within functions with experienced project managers, valuable generic plans can be developed. These can be customized to specific projects. Obviously every project is unique; however, there are many common "building blocks" that need to be put in place for projects of a similar type. To create "generic" plans it is necessary to establish a limited number of project "types" with clearly stated basis of assumptions. This enables the cross-functional cycle time reduction team to reexamine the activities that need to be conducted and how they need to be sequenced. Best estimates of activity durations are reviewed. The dependencies for initiation of activities can be challenged. What exactly does the "draft report" have to contain? The exercise is valuable in fostering a better understanding of how functional contributions fit into the overall delivery of the project. By some creative cross-functional thinking, time-saving options will be found and by iterative interrogation of the plan, time-saving strategies will be found. Generally, a balance point is reached when it becomes clear that two or more major lines of activity are on or are very close to the critical path for the project and further attempts to achieve cycle time reduction will bring only modest time saving but an appreciable increase in the risk of failure.

In past times, the duration of a development project generally was dictated by the duration of the clinical program. This was because the conduct of clinical trials and their reporting out (particularly the time taken from database lock of phase 3 trials to the availability of integrated efficacy and safety summaries) was quite protracted. As a result of process improvement and electronic data capture and analysis, clinical operations and database management is now a much slicker enterprise. As a result, the critical path pressure is often on other groups notably CMC and long-term toxicology (refer to chaps. 3 and 4).

An important by-product of such process improvement initiatives is the resultant closer collaboration of line functions with project management. Functions are sensitive about being rate-limiting to projects and keen to understand how their deliverables fit into the time lines. This has promoted the adoption of project planning systems within functions as smart functional managers recognized the benefits to the efficient management of their groups. This in turn led to within-function cycle time reduction initiatives that identified ways of reducing delivery time that could be fed back into the "whole project" plans. Clinical and regulatory functions were able to find appreciable time savings to the delivery of their key "products."

Cycle time reduction initiatives create valuable understanding between project management and line functions of the extent of the interdependency of development work, to provide a platform to challenge the status quo of "how we do things here" and to establish "benchmark" generic plans. Benchmark plans help senior managers to more intelligently interrogate project time lines.

ACQUIRING THE SKILLS FOR THE JOB

Using a Competency Framework

Training needs should be reviewed in an open discussion between the manager and the job holder against a competency framework. This discussion should identify the most important areas for development of skills and competencies. For each competency, the organization describes the required (i) basic level, (ii) intermediate level, and (iii) superior level. Feedback should be gathered from a few experienced team members on the perceived competency level prior to a review meeting with the manager.

The feedback should be reviewed and the discussion can then focus on those areas where there is agreement that development to the next level is required in order to accomplish the new tasks.

Competency frameworks should not become leaden, bureaucratic constructs. It is up to the organization to judge what should be the standards required and then to select training interventions as appropriate.

General Management Skills

To lead an IPT effectively, the team leader must have excellent general management skills. Some pharma companies have established training programs in collaboration with top international business schools. In some cases, specific pharma-related training programs have been established. There are a number of important skills that a team leader needs to deploy. These skills are now discussed.

Communications Skills

It is difficult to resist the temptation to become totally immersed in the technical details of a project and in doing so lose sight of the big picture and core objectives. Dealing with complexity and reducing it to simpler value propositions is the essence of good management. Clarity is valued. Communications skills are vital for an effective team leader. Recognizing who the stakeholders are, understanding their agenda and their needs, and making the time for individual briefings in advance of major presentations discriminate the effective team leaders. Their passion for the project translates into actions to bring stakeholders on board. It is particularly important to understand that there are often a number of communication vehicles that need to be used to ensure that the project's "message" is understood within the company at large and within the functions. Typically, the team leader will present a new development plan in conjunction with a request for resources to support the implementation of the plan for the next 18 months. The pharma board reviews and sanctions the request. The presentation to this committee and the supporting documentation precirculated to the review committee are important components in the decision process. But for many projects in mid-phase development, a variety of issues and uncertainties exist. It is essential that the project team leader has open channels of communication with functional heads to ensure that there is a shared understanding of the risks even if there persists a difference in perception of the magnitude of the risk. For the review committee, it will be readily apparent when the team leader has had the maturity to engage with a function to try to get to a joint understanding of risk and when a blinkered "we know best" approach has been adopted. Presentation skills are important to the team leader and can be developed. Some companies have tackled this by providing internal training with coaching and demonstration sessions often with film recording so that the participants can witness the impact of their presentations and the areas for improvement. In addition, there some excellent external training programs that get to the heart of communication strategy. Jerry Weissman's training program is excellent (1)

Negotiation Skills

The team leader and project managers can benefit from training in negotiation skills. While it is not their job generally to be negotiating contracts (though this may well be the case in smaller biotech companies), the awareness of negotiation techniques is valuable. There are invariably a range of contentious issues that occur during the project history. It is easy for the issues to degenerate into partisan positions that owe more to the conflicting personalities than to the problem to be addressed. Training in negotiating skills can provide a structured approach to problem resolution and help people gain more confidence by understanding the boundaries in negotiation and how to work with other parties to achieve the best outcome.

Problem Solving and Decision Analysis

If negotiating skills are important so is the quality of problem analysis. Some companies have tackled the latter by broad organizational training programs so that when "decision analysis" is mentioned there is an immediate understanding of the processes that will be applied. One example of this is the Kepner-Tregoe program, which provides superb case study examples of woeful decision making as a backdrop to setting a robust process for companies to use (2). The emphasis on the importance of being clear on the decision objectives is particularly valuable.

Business Skills

While some team leaders and project manager have business qualifications, they are a minority. Most development and project management people have scientific backgrounds. As a result, the perspective of team leaders tends to be technical and scientific rather than a commercial or business perspective. This is an important issue because ultimately drug development is a business that delivers commercial products at an investment risk. Some companies have tackled this radically by transferring leadership responsibility for late-stage projects to the global strategic marketing group to ensure a strong commercial focus. Other approaches include secondment of team leaders to central or national marketing groups to gain a better understanding of what is needed to promote product use in a territory and the critical importance of product-labeling that can be exploited commercially. Several commercial programs offer training in marketing, pricing and re-imbursement, pharmacoeconomics, project valuation methodology and deal strategy. In addition, some Business Schools including INSEAD have established Pharma focused business training programs.

Drug Development Skills

On-the-job learning
The intellectual caliber of people working in development in our industry is invariably high and this is one factor in why it is a rewarding working environment. Smart people watch, listen, and learn with amazing speed. Just participating in project team meetings for a novice is a stimulating experience and, initially, somewhat intimidating since there are a lot of unfamiliar acronyms flying round, the principles of development are unfamiliar, and your team members are unknown quantities. However, in the first six months of participation on the team, the learning curve is prodigious even without specific training programs. The background of the "novice" may help the transition. For example, there is a flow of people who have worked in multidisciplinary discovery projects who decide that they would

like their further career to be in development. Such individuals bring with them an understanding of several of the scientific disciplines supporting development.

Mentoring

Mentoring potentially is probably one of the best ways of training new project management staff. In many professions, the practice of an "apprentice" working alongside the "master" to learn a trade has endured. It works well today provided that the mentor is both highly capable and fully committed to the role. A high-caliber project manager or project leader deploys a range of skills appropriate to the setting and has a broad understanding of development principles and strategies likely gained in the management of a number of development projects over the years. The novice, therefore, will see how the team leader works with the team, how expert contributions are drawn out, how open discussion is encouraged to get the best creativity from team members in addressing project issues, and how such creativity is then translated into clearly defined actions. The communication, negotiation, and interpersonal skills of the team leader can be seen in action. In addition, while during a project team meeting there might be insufficient time for the novice to fully understand issues in discussion but after the meeting, a debrief will allow for a full discussion and often "war stories" of similar issues encountered on other projects that the team leader has led.

Assignments

During the first 18 months in the project management group, valuable learning experience can be gained from well-planned assignments. A newcomer will recognize in the quality of their personal development plan that the company values them and is intelligently aiming to equip them with the skills they need. In addition to being delegated to be a member of a particular project team for a reasonable period, it is valuable for shorter assignments during which there is a chance to become better acquainted with the business. In some cases, these may be well-organized visits, for example, to a production facility organized by the manufacturing project team member during which the manufacturing process and quality control processes can be seen in action. In some cases, it may be two days work shadowing clinical operations staff in planning a clinical trial. The learning opportunities in such assignments are considerable if the project manager is keen to learn and the accepting group is committed. The chance of the latter is greater if there is a reciprocal program.

Seminar series

A rolling seminar series is a great way of tapping into the knowledge and expertise within a pharmaceutical company and sharing this across the organization. A good way of developing a drug development series is to develop a consistent format for presentations for each of the key disciplines in development. A project management group can take the initiative to set up the series by giving the first seminar, which would be a "development overview" describing the phases of development, the structure of project teams, and the scope of the work activities carried out to register a drug. This seminar would be followed by presentations from clinical, toxicology, drug metabolism, scale chemistry, formulation, regulatory, pharmacoeconomics, marketing, and so on. There is upfront work in the creation of the slide packs but once this is done, the seminar series can run at different company sites and by different presenters from the discipline departments. These seminars are well received and often run over the lunch break. The presentations can easily be converted to a "notes" format that can be given to the participants with a concise narrative.

Simulation training programs

A few companies have established drug development training programs that use simulation techniques to give course participants the chance to "develop" a drug in a controlled environment that permits assessment and expert feedback. This type of training program demands a significant investment in time and resource to set up. However, there is no doubt that it is highly effective in giving participants a good insight into development strategy and the nature of drug development. To establish a drug development simulation training program, a case study is first constructed. This involves the creation of a background package of information and data for the drug, which provides the participating teams a number of potential clinical indications. The teams comprise the usual project team disciplines. The teams establish TPPs for each indication. A development activities database is provided to the teams together with a planning tool. Teams build their project plans and can see the time and cost of the development of the indications. The preferred development strategy is selected that may involve decision not to develop some indications, parallel or staggered or sequential development strategies. A faculty reviews and approves the "plans." This part of the program takes about two days and introduces many people for the first time to the multiple factors that need to be considered in selecting the best strategy and the critical importance that the TPP plays in setting the plan. The plan is then implemented in simulation with the years of development collapsed into a couple of days. Results from each development activity in each discipline are released as each activity is completed. A variety of "problems" are designed into a selection of the activities. This requires teams firstly to recognize that a problem has indeed been encountered and then to propose a viable solution. At the end of the plan implementation, the teams present their development plan as proposed for implementation and as it turned out in implementation to a faculty review group. There is a great opportunity to involve the senior management of the drug company at this stage. This is really appreciated by the team members who rarely have the chance to meet and hear the top team. The top team also evidently enjoys the opportunity to visit the team rooms, meet team members, and see the work in progress on the Thursday afternoon as teams finalize their presentations. The review of the team plans provides a great way of capturing the lessons of the week and teams hear the critiques of the executives from discovery, development, and marketing. An additional feature of this sort of program is that of teamwork. The program is highly intensive and somewhat stressful as the teams have never worked together before and many have not been in real project teams before. Faculties need therefore to monitor the progress of each team carefully as from time to time some coaching is needed. While establishing and running a simulation training program is demanding in time and resource, the participants in such programs invariably judge them to be amongst the strongest training programs that they have experienced. The internal reputation of these programs means that a queue rapidly builds up of people wanting to enroll. Figure 4 depicts the way that drug simulation training can be run.

Reading schemes
Today it is easy to access quickly the available literature on any subject and, depending on the search engine and search strategy, to identify articles and books that are of value. The reader review assessments are very useful to discriminate the disparity between book title "advert" and text "value." There is a copious literature on project management but a very limited literature specifically focused on pharmaceutical project management. There are a lot of books on drug development including the extensive series "Drugs and the Pharmaceutical Sciences" published by Marcel Dekker of which the first edition of this book was Volume 86. A few informative books have been published on drug development which are worth reading because the scope of the text is broad and relevant and the authorship is expert (3, 4, 5).

Professional societies
There are a few pharmaceutical industry project management groups that organize meetings for their membership and maintain links with the international community. In Europe, the Pharmaceutical Industry Project Management Group (PIPMG), established in 1985, organizes meetings twice a year and actively fosters links with related professional societies. The reader is encouraged to go to their site for helpful links to a number of other organizations that provide training either in drug development or project management (6).

The European Center of Pharmaceutical Medicine in Basel offers postgraduate training in pharmaceutical medicine, which is aimed at scientists involved in drug development. Six sessions of three or four days' duration that are run over two years cover a broad range of development topics including one devoted to "project and product management." The faculty includes acknowledgement experts in their fields (7).

A similar program is now run in the United States of America with an inaugural cycle commencing in September 2007. The course is titled "The American Course on Drug Development and Regulatory Sciences" and has been constructed with the involvement of academic, industry, and FDA experts. One session is focused on integrated product development strategy, execution, and project management and is led by highly experienced chairpersons (8).

In the United States, the Pharmaceutical Education and Research Institute (PERI) offers a number of drug development programs including a three-day program titled "Project Management in the Research-Based Pharmaceutical Industry."

In the United Kingdom, Management Forum has for many years run a successful two-day training program "Project Management for Pharmaceutical Professionals" (9).

REFERENCES

1. Weissman J. Presenting to Win. Financial Times Prentice Hall, New Jersey, USA, 2003.
2. Kepner-Tregoe. www.kepner-tregoe.com
3. Welling, Lasagna and Banaker. The Drug Development Process. Volume 76 in the Drugs and the Pharmaceutical Sciences, Marcel Dekker, New York, USA, 1996.
4. Edwards L, Fletcher A, Fox A, et al. Principles and Practice of Pharmaceutical Medicine 2nd edn. Wiley, UK, 2007.
5. Evens R. Drug and Biological Development, Springer, USA, 2007.
6. Pharmaceutical Industry Project Management Group (PIPMG) website. www.pipmg. org/training_industry_links.htm.
7. The European Center of Pharmaceutical Medicine website. www.ecpm.ch
8. The American Course on Drug Development and Regulatory Sciences site. http://acdrs.ucsf.edu
9. Management Forum training program in Pharmaceutical Project Management. info@management-forum.co.uk

Index